The Keto Edge

Keto Secrets That Change Your Body, Your Health,
Your Future, and Your Life!

———————

David M. Woynarowski, M.D.,
Oksana Zagorodna, Ph.D.

Internal Alchemy Press.com Publisher

Disclaimer: This book is written for people who do not have diabetes or any other abnormality that would affect their blood sugar or handling of ketones in an adverse fashion such as kidney disease. You should get a complete physical exam and consult your personal physician before attempting a ketogenic diet. Only attempt this diet if you are healthy and non-diabetic.

Please read the chapter notes carefully if you are diabetic. If you are requiring insulin to control your blood sugars or have a long (greater than 2-year) history of diabetes, especially if you are poorly controlled, do not attempt these diets without direct medical supervision. Ketogenic diets are potentially very beneficial in the early stages of diabetes and pre-diabetes but only if the individual is aware of the proper way to administer this diet. Similarly, the weight loss and saluresis (kidney getting rid of salt) can be very beneficial for those with high blood pressure, if the particulars of the diet are followed.

Please note: No medical claims are made, suggested, insinuated or otherwise advanced by this book. No claims of disease prevention, diagnosis, mitigation, or cure are made. The user assumes all responsibility for the use, misuse, or non-use of the information provided here which is for informational purposes only.

Dedication

This book is dedicated to the brilliant everyday individuals who choose to savor their life's journey in making each meal exquisitely healthy and simply delicious.

table of contents

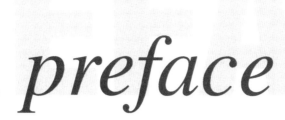

preface

The idea for this book started way back in 2012. It holds as true today as it did then. At the time I was horrified at what I call the "Business of Cancer". The Business of Cancer refers to the traditional medical view of cancer as a disease and how a huge industry of paraphernalia, behavior and inaccuracies about progress were being sold to and consumed by the public by the Medical Industrial Complex which I had been a part of.

Then, as now, the statistics surrounding this disease are often massaged to give a more optimistic view of the progress medical science has made. The death rate for cancer, especially metastatic cancer, has changed very little since President Nixon declared war on the disease in 1970. Survival rates that were originally measured in 10-year increments dropped to 5 years, and now claims of "extending life" are made when less than a year is added to survival.

Simply put, as obvious as it sounds, cancer remains now, as then, a disease that is better not to get.

Dr. Zagorodna and I had read a book called "Cancer as a Metabolic Disease," by Dr. Tom Seyfried, Ph.D. Calorie-restricted ketogenic diet was discussed to have potential as either an alternative or additional modality to treat or prevent cancer. At the time, Dr. Zagorodna was working in cancer prevention and metabolic cancer research at MD Anderson Cancer Center and later at Baylor College of Medicine. The information in the book was invaluable to both Oksana's work in advancing the existing cancer prevention/treatments strategies, and to my outlook from the clinical perspective. We have been more aware of both research and clinical implications while individually exploring the benefits of the Keto approach for human health.

Keto diets are defined as very low carbohydrate intake and very high fat intake.

The simple question to ask was: How feasible is it to go on this kind of diet (Keto) for a healthy person, let alone a person with cancer? Dr. Seyfried's compelling scientific arguments drew me into the experiment on myself.

Could healthy persons implement and benefit from the Keto diet, and was it possible to then recommend this diet to people suffering from cancer or other diseases?

The answer turned out to be "YES!" but, this is not a book about cancer.

In the years that followed until now, Keto would become the next craze and a popularly adopted lifestyle approach.

From my personal experience, I can say that the near magical changes in my appearance, my blood chemistries, and my energy levels spawned a long-term lifestyle change that I continue to this day.

In addition, the science has finally caught up with the diet, and so many misrepresentations and unfounded fears have been replaced with research that backs up the safety and health-giving properties of this diet.

Even more compelling to me as an Anti-Aging and Regenerative Medicine doctor are the potential improvements from the diet on Health Span (how much of your life is spent in good health) and Life Span.

In this book, we share with you the theoretical and practical Keto approaches that we have learned and applied along the way!

~ Dave Woynarowski, M.D. (Pennsylvania, 2020)

acknowledgements

First and foremost, I would like to express gratitude to my colleague, Dr. Oksana Zagorodna. Oksana's indispensable collaboration has contributed scientifically to all that I have reviewed clinically to yield "The Keto Edge" book. Our shared curiosity on Ketogenic diet summarizes theory and practice of Keto with the goal to advance human Health Span (how much of your life is spent in good health) throughout Life Span.

Our in-depth Keto explorations were enriched from reading Tom Seyfried's book "Cancer as a Metabolic Disease." In addition to reading his book, I had the pleasure of spending many hours dialoguing with Tom. I appreciated our Keto conversations, the numerous questions that were asked and answered, and the advanced knowledge on the Keto subject.

To the brilliant minds who have stimulated mine and continue to do so, Rafael Gonzalez Ph.D., Maria Blasco, Ph.D., Bill Lands, Ph.D., Luis Daniel Ortega, Ph.D., Michael Fossel, M.D., Ph.D., my co-author of The Immortality Edge (along with Greta Blackburn, another pioneer in the field) and an inspirational worker in the field of Anti-Aging and Longevity.

To Dr. Bill Andrews, Ph.D., who co-discovered the human telomerase gene. Thanks for making aging optional, Bill, and for all your sharing of knowledge and insights. How lucky I have been to have been with such exceptional minds!

To my current crop of students, friends, and people who obviously care – I hope my work keeps you young and healthy!

To Dr. Robert Atkins, M.D., who popularized his version of Keto over 40 years ago and began the fire that started the modern Keto Revolution. I was in my teens then and – believe it or not – spent a half a year experimenting with that diet. Predictably, I lost over 20 pounds, most of it fat, and became a poster child for the shredded look!

And finally, last but absolutely not least, my original and continued mentor, Matt Furey – how appreciative I am to know you, how fortunate I was to meet you, and how wise of both of us to transcend the slings and arrows of everyday life and remain in contact for all these many years, each of us growing younger by the day! I remain your mostly student, rarely teacher, and always friend!

Because of all of you – the Magic Continues!

Dave Woynarowski, M.D.

introduction

The goal of this book is to provide you with an in-depth knowledge of the way Keto works in your body and to give you specific recipes as tools to achieve ketosis and maintain it without sacrificing the delicious experience of food!

This book is a result of many hours in research and review to assist you, the reader, in understanding the science behind the ketogenic meals every step of the way, as you venture in creating your own Keto favorites!

We have featured specific active ingredients in each recipe to highlight what can be truly beneficial, rather than just tasting good, all the while helping you stay in ketosis.

You don't have to be a scientist to understand this book, but it will help if you are curious! This book will benefit the most those who wish to know "why" things work the way they do.

Of course, if you just want to dive into great tasting recipes, you can always jump right to that section and get started!

That said, going Keto is greatly helped if you understand how to use this knowledge way beyond the recipes. We include a lot of tips and detailed descriptions of what the metabolic changes are doing to you and how you will feel when they happen. Ketogenic effects become maximally beneficial if the diet is practiced using ecologically clean, nutritious products.

Knowing the science behind Keto diet has made the experience a lot easier, less frightening, and has given better results to our beta testers all of whom are not scientists!

the original ancestral diet

Ketogenic Diet transcends human history.

Ketogenic diet was here before we could speak in sentences. It was here before we lived in cities, raised animals and crops, and had extended families. It was here when humans were hunter-gatherers and lived in small mobile tribes and communities that spent most of their time looking for food.

The main reason Ketogenic lifestyle is so useful and healthful for us now is because it was likely a mainstay of our eating during the formative times of our genetic code. You may have heard the term "Space aged minds in Stone Aged bodies" used to describe people of today. This is actually accurate.

Almost all of the things that are written into our genetic code were completed between 50,000 and 200,000 years ago.

Human history is very short compared to other species on the planet. In the grand scheme of how we evolve, it takes hundreds of millions of years for major changes to occur.

The same is not true of us as a culture! In the past hundred years we have changed so dramatically that our immediate ancestors do not recognize what we have become. Nothing illustrates this more than our diet.

But before we get into that, let's journey back in time. Let's go back about 50,000 years. Our ancestors were hunter-gatherers and faced what we would consider extraordinary challenges in eating, finding, and storing food. Fortunately, we were endowed with equally extraordinary adaptability.

The ancestral "you and I" likely went without food for several hours, or even days at a time. Thus, the concept of fasting was born not of civilization or religion, but of necessity. If we could not fast, we would not have survived as a species. Since our genes – and in particular those genes that pertain to food and nutrition – were "born and shaped" during this time, fasting is a natural healthy process even now.

Along with fasting comes ketosis.

What is ketosis? In very simple terms, it refers to the body's ability to do without *carbohydrates* (carbs), and to burn stored fat as the primary fuel. While carbohydrate is the sprint-like immediate source of energy, fat is the form of energy we store for the long haul.

Ketosis digs into fat mass and burns it, recycling a lot of garbage we have stored in the fatty tissues and allowing our body to 'run clean.'

As we consume stored fats, we shift our eating to consume more fats and to avoid carbohydrates. For our purposes, carbohydrates should be easy to identify: they include added sugars (total grams of sugar per serving size should be less than 10 grams, and YES you do have to watch the serving size).

Carbohydrate-containing food includes all sugared beverages, breads, pastas and starchy vegetables like potatoes. Theoretically, you could eat some of these things, as long as you kept your total carbohydrate intake below 50 grams per day. It is important to note that carbohydrate grams add up very fast. For example, one slice of bread can range from 35 to 100 grams of carbs.

High levels of carbohydrate consumption lead to the rise, followed by the drop, in insulin and blood sugar. Even if the sugar levels do not go above normal in your blood stream, the rise and subsequent fall will cause you to be more hungry and have a much harder time eating fewer carbs in your next meal. Simply put, you will crave carbs if you eat a lot of them!

The presence or absence of sugar and carbohydrates in our diet is the main determinant of whether or not we are in ketosis. Our bodies respond to sugar, or more specifically to carbohydrates, by secreting a hormone called *insulin*. While the complete actions of insulin are beyond the scope of this book, insulin is – first and foremost – a FAT STORAGE hormone.

In the absence of insulin, your body cannot store any significant amount of fat.

Let's go back to the "ancestral you and me" again.

Our ancestors were lean, muscular and very very healthy and strong by today's standards. And they were disease free. They were lean primarily because of their diet. They had a much higher daily intake of fat and protein and a much lower intake of carbohydrates.

Let's look at these statements individually.

Our ancestors were muscular. It is hard to fathom the muscularity of our ancestors compared to the average person these days. Now, of course, they were far more active than we are. There were no desks, chairs, or automobiles to carry them to and from places. Our ancestors moved only under their own power. But the actual muscularity was, and even is, not just a function of exercise. There are millions of people who go to the gym and do what they think is proper exercise, getting very little of the desired result from it.

In almost every case this is because of diet. Today's fascination with "Six Pack Abs" has bombarded everyone! It has spawned billion-dollar industries that focus on machines and gadgets to give us the look of muscularity that our ancestors had, primarily because of their ketogenic diets.

While this is not a book on aesthetics, one of the side benefits of maintaining the high fat ketogenic diet is that your body will transform into a lean and muscular appearance faster than any gadget or even any exercise plan could ever give you.

Our ancestors didn't care about any of this!

They did not care about six packs or pecs or "getting big." They just wanted to eat and made choices about their calorie sources that would maximize their survival and health. They were, as we shall see, more or less forced into a higher fat ketogenic low carb diet by nature and by their own genetic makeup.

But they were ripped, lean, and muscular as a result! They would, no doubt, be astounded at how we look as a species today!

In those days, our ancestors were strong. In truth, only the strong survived. Our ancestors had to move, work, and hunt almost every day. Some days they were successful and others not – hence the need to be able to survive periods of fasting.

The type of work and hunting they did often involved long periods of endurance interspersed with explosive strength. If you want the perfect exercise program, model your fitness plans in that fashion. In addition, remember they did not have gyms, barbells, kettle bells or elliptical orbiters! They ran, they jumped, they climbed and used primarily their body weight.

Our ancestors were healthy! Archeological and paleobiologic studies of our ancestors revealed that while they did not live long lives (30 was more common than 40!), they did not suffer from chronic ailments to the degree that we do.

Now, it is true they did not have the time to develop those ailments, as "old age" was probably 40 years old for them. By far, the most common cause of death was trauma-based. That would include traumatic childbirth, trauma from hunting, and infections from trauma incurred during daily life.

In summary, our ancestors' lives were shorter, more desperate and violent than ours, and mainly centered on food gathering for survival.

But what kind of food? Well pretty much everything or anything that they could hunt or forage for.

The work of Loren Cordain, Ph.D. and others suggests that our ancestors ate a lot more fat and protein than we do today.

Remember, they did not grow crops but foraged for plants and nuts, and to a far lesser extent grains. If you think of the amount of nutrition and calories that could be had and how many mouths could be fed from killing a deer or two versus finding a berry patch, you will understand why necessity forced them to focus on fat and protein over carbohydrates.

Next, let's take the special case of "The Hunt".

Ancient culture is difficult to define because of the lack of written records and large clusters of fossils. But groups of more than fifty or a hundred people living in one spot together were rare. Finding the fossil records of those tribes is very difficult.

One thing is for certain – whether our ancestors were roaming the desert sands or the frozen tundra, they were hunting for survival.

The meat and fat they hunted provided food not only for themselves, but for the rest of their tribe or group. It is difficult to overstress the importance of the hunt in ancient society as a social determinant and a survival determinant. But along with all that, our human ancestors were being shaped in terms of what they would pass on to us with regards to our nutritional needs.

They were carnivores whenever they could be and herbivores when they had to be. Often, they were the ultimate Flexitarians!

Even more so, they were the benefactors, victims and arbiters of their diet. And their central struggle to find food as a life or death issue shaped the changes in human diets that followed!

We, contemporary humans, have their genes from 50,000 to 200,000 years ago. We have not only the ability to live on a high fat diet, but the actual need for lower carbs and higher fat with some protein, because of who they were and what they did.

When they hunted, they had to carry their food after they caught it. Studies of modern hunter-gatherer tribes that have kept at least some of the old ways alive, as well as studies from those types of tribes that survived long enough to have their habits documented (Pacific Northwest Native Americans and Eskimos), tell us that they lived on fat as the primary fuel source, especially during the hunt.

Once again, since a Flexitarian lifestyle is what most of our ancestors spent their time doing, it is the very makeup of what we are as human biologic machines. We store fat when we can. We burn fat almost every second of the day. Our sub-cellular powerhouses known as mitochondria are like little furnaces that burn fat mixed with oxygen as a primary fuel source. Fat contributes greatly to a healthy energetic lifestyle.

necessity is the mother of invention and the father of change – good or bad!

A fundamental change in society and human behavior started to happen 10,000 to 15,000 years ago. We as a species started to favor living in larger and larger groups with less and less tendency to move and hunt for our food. This was made possible by the ability to grow crops and raise domesticated farm animals. The exact dawn of the agricultural age of man is not known, but its impact on our metabolism is clear.

We adapted to living in larger groups and to having a man-made infrastructure. The primary result of this was we were able to remain stationary instead of roaming the land and hunting.

The specifics of what we ate changed radically from wild game and foraged plants, nuts, seeds, and insects to the types of grains and meats we eat now. The farmer, not the hunter, became responsible for feeding the village.

The cultivation of grains, in particular, led to a significant increase and even, some might say, a dependency on carbohydrates for a major portion of our calories. Milling and baking were developed as technologies to release the nutrients in grain-based foods, further changing their position in our diets from background to the major food source.

Of course, fasting – both enforced from climatic variations and for religious reasons – continued, but the fundamental makeup of society and the foods we eat changed seemingly forever!

From a developmental and nutritional standpoint, this posed some metabolic problems that we are just now beginning to understand at various levels including genetics. Genetic changes are very slow to occur in most cases.

We did not exactly have time to adapt to the so-called modern carb-based diet. We were forged in the hunter gatherer mold and not the farmer mold; as a result, while we may live longer, we now face diseases of "old age".

In strictly scientific terms, it is hard to link diseases of old age directly with our diet. However, as time goes on, the high carbohydrate diets of the past century become the suggested causes of obesity, diabetes, heart disease, and even cancer!

Other factors, such as activity levels and social environment, as well as lifestyle choices, are now factors in how we live, whereas they were not so before. Before, finding food was the main thing. Now, it has descended greatly on most people's list.

The most obvious result of all this change is that as a species most humans make a lot more insulin than their ancestors did, because they consume a lot more carbohydrates.

Paleontologists estimate that our hunter-gatherer ancestors ate somewhere between 50 and 100 grams of carbs daily depending on where they lived. Right now, the average person on a store-bought western diet consumes 3 to 5X that amount and thus makes 3 to 5X as much insulin. Add to this the increased portion sizes and, in some cultures, the routine consumption of fermented grain drinks in the form of alcohol, and you will see that, for some, these estimates are likely to be low.

No one has ever looked specifically or singly at the long-term effects of a diet that contains 500 or more grams of carbohydrates daily. But in the short run, getting fat and having insulin issues are clearly demonstrated.

As we study aging and the diseases of aging, we begin to understand the role of excess insulin in damaging our bodies. Insulin, the fat storage hormone, can, when it is made in excess, become a source of inflammation in our body. So, too, can the increased fat stores that accompany it.

Without getting deeply into biochemistry, fat is an active organ that makes (secretes) chemical messengers.

When fat storage is present in excess amounts, our bodies become inflamed, and this accelerates the aging process. We also become obese or simply overweight. Please notice the text did not say "when fat is consumed in large amounts"!

Obesity has also been linked to cancer, diabetes, heart disease and arthritis, to name but a few of the diseases of "old age" that we see more and more of.

The simple fundamental change of going back to more of an ancestral diet is a valuable one for our health and longevity.

Now the question is: What parts of the ancestral diet should we focus on?

If we try to imitate as best we can what our ancestors ate, it becomes obsessive and impractical. Currently, there is a Paleo Diet movement that has gained a lot of followers.

Alongside that dietary habit is the rise of a specific type of exercise called "Crossfit" TM. Both of these disciplines attempt to make the combination of diet and exercise closely fitting with what our ancestors did.

While certainly meritorious, as each has grown to have millions of followers, the basic principles have been heavily diluted for mass consumption.

The simplest form of Paleo diet is worth looking at, since it does mirror some principles of the Ketogenic diet. Avoiding dairy (not a ketogenic principle) and avoiding grain (definitely a ketogenic principle) are the tenants of this diet. The idea is that ancestral hunter-gatherer societies were not raising dairy animals or practicing agriculture, thus these food groups are to be avoided.

This diet works very well for many people and is useful in between ketogenic diet periods if you are not interested in, or capable of, maintaining a long term ketogenic diet, or you happen to be lactose and/or gluten intolerant.

The main difference between Paleo diets and ketogenic diets, of course, is the state of ketosis. Our ancestors had to deal with long periods of fasting, sometimes days or even weeks. Because few sources of concentrated carbohydrates actually existed for daily consumption, it is just as likely that our ancestors were in ketosis for long periods of time.

Ketosis only happens for most people when they are significantly carbohydrate restricted.

The magic number of 50 grams a day seems to be a good starting place for a ketogenic diet. For reference, this amount of carbs is about the same as in 1 and ½ slices of bread. Keep in mind that most foods are not totally carbohydrate free. So, before you gobble the 1 and ½ slices of bread for breakfast, thinking you will avoid carbs the rest of the day, be advised that is not going to happen. Even sugarless gum has 2 grams of carbs per 2-piece serving size.

An ideal way to get into ketosis is to superimpose it onto a fast. Fasting for 18 hours a day, then consuming a moderately sized meal consisting of mostly fat and some protein is an ideal way to do this. Note that this means some favorites have to go. Fruits in particular have to be limited.

Because of the dehydrated and concentrated nature of dates, one or two dates will put you close to the limit. For standard fruits like apples, pears, oranges, it is ok to eat half of one daily.

Most of your fiber, vitamins and minerals will come from green leafy vegetables. Again, to maximize the benefit, you should stick with kale, spinach, cabbage, broccoli, and darker more robust forms of lettuce (not iceberg lettuce!). These are low in calories and carbs, but are high in nutrition.

terms, facts and fallacies – so you won't get fooled again!

It can be useful to know the terms and definitions that are frequently used in Keto literature.

Let's start with *The Glycemic Index:* The Glycemic Index (GI) is a tool often used by dieters and dieticians alike to determine the "impact" of sugars in a certain food. The food's impact on a person's blood sugar (how fast or slow a food enters the bloodstream and raises your blood sugar level) is compared to an impact by a standard, which is usually pure glucose consumed in the same amount. Generally, foods with high GI are best to be avoided. Pure glucose is considered "100" (mg/dL), and everything else is compared to it. Note that this is not sucrose or table sugar, which, ironically, is considered a "medium glycemic index food" with a number between 50 and 69.

The Glycemic Load: The Glycemic Load (GL) is the impact a food has on a person's blood sugar when compared to consumption of 1 gram of glucose. While neither of these measurements is perfect for our purposes, it is reasonable to stick to lower glycemic index foods consumed in quantities that do not exceed the amounts normally listed as portion sizes.

This becomes important because things like grain derived foods, especially processed cereals, often come in as "medium" glycemic load foods. But their portion sizes are often listed as ¼ to ½ cup which would not satisfy your cat! In this way it is deceptive to look at labels. Always look at portion sizes and see if they are indeed acceptable.

Similarly, a cup of red raspberries is listed as 13 grams of carbs, which, while not excessive, is not a little amount either! But most of us would be satisfied with less than a cup, or certainly no more.

Cherries, figs (if not dehydrated) and most other berries are great lower carb sources of phytopigments (coloring matter in plants that gives them their color) that contain many antioxidants.

As mentioned above, dates are out of the picture. One single date runs you about 18 grams of carbs, that means with 3 or 4 of them you are over your daily limit!

In dealing with the Glycemic Load: think of this as the actual number of carbs/sugars you are consuming, so it takes into account your portion sizes (with an emphasis on "your"). If you have a cookie that is low in glycemic index, but you eat a dozen of them, your glycemic load is going to be high no matter what!

We do have several dessert recipes in this book, so keep in mind that portion control is still a key point when you are consuming desserts!

There is a lot of debate about using these measurements, because there are some high protein foods that can cause a fair amount of *insulin* because of their protein content. You have to resort to something called the *Insulin Index* to find these things out. If you are into numbers, consider looking into the Insulin Index, as well, to use it in your daily calorie/carb calculations.

The bottom line is: if you stick with the calorie % breakdown of 60 to 70% fat, 20% protein and 10% carbs, your totals will not need to be calculated.

You will be in ketosis!

Staying away from high glycemic index food may be the simplest and best way to keep things where you want them. As a general rule, most melons (watermelon in small amounts is an exception because of the water content), grapes, pineapples, mangoes, and papayas are all off the list for regular consumption.

By saying regular consumption, it is suggested that once in a while you might indulge, but be aware of the following: *Ketogenic diets are easiest to maintain when you do not indulge.* Sugar is addictive, and a seemingly small indulgence can open the floodgates to much larger transgressions. Also, be advised: it does not take much of an indulgence to bump you out of ketosis!

In summary, stick with the calorie percentages for fats, proteins and carbs, and you will not have to worry about much else. This is especially true if you are calorie restricting the way we recommend.

Two great ways to calorie-restrict are: a 3-day water-only fast (you can add in bouillon if need be for the salt) and a 7 to 14 day calorie restriction of 500 calories or less.

It will take your body a minimum of 2 to 3 days to go into full ketosis no matter what you do.

How will you know that you are in ketosis?

The best ways to tell are to actually document this.

One way to document is by collecting the data from a blood fingerstick. The medical device company Abbott makes a glucose-ketone meter, and you can measure both blood sugar and ketones with a basically painless fingerstick. Sadly, these measurements are not cheap because the ketone strips cost about $5 US apiece.

Many people will opt for the entirely satisfactory measure of using a urine ketone strip. These ketone strips are far less precise when it comes to quantitating the *amount* of ketones in your body, but they do document the presence or absence of ketones. Since most people do not fast long enough to have ANY ketones present, a positive urine strip is telling you that you are going in the right direction.

If you do opt to use blood strips, be aware there are different degrees of ketosis:

Borderline ketosis: Anything between 0.1 and 1.5 mmol/L is considered borderline. You will be getting the benefits of ketosis but not quite to the optimal level of them.

Optimal level ketosis: The optimal level usually occurs between 1.5 and 3.5 mmol/L as measured by a blood fingerstick device. Keep in mind that most of these devices may be calibrated for USA use (if you get them through mailing order), so the numbers may be different in the UK or Europe. In the UK, optimal levels of ketones will be between 0.6 mmol/L and 1.6 mmol/L. The number you should look for depends on which measurement your meter reads, which will, in turn, be determined by where you bought it!

Just a quick side note before you get into the actual recipes. This book was originally started in 2012, and some definitions have changed: 50 grams of daily carbohydrate dose is used as a cutoff to achieve ketosis, because this is what we have seen in personal dieting to accommodate ketosis. The definition has now changed: the "moderately low carb" levels are at 50 grams of daily carbohydrate intake, while the "low carb" cutoff is at 20 grams.

From Dr. Dave's personal experience:

> When I first went Keto in 2012, I used to check my ketones and blood sugars with a fingerstick monitor. I routinely hit a nice 4 mmol/L measurement, with blood sugars in the 30-40 mg/dL range with no symptoms of low blood sugar.

I have found after time that the urine dipsticks are reasonably good and reflect the relative amount of ketones in your blood, even though it's a urine test. For most people, I do not see the need to measure blood ketones. Keep in mind: when you use exogenous ketone drinks like my Keto Gen, you will see normal blood sugars, even though your ketones are higher than normal.

Some Terms to Watch Out For:

Low Carb: Currently defined as consuming less than 20 grams of carbs per day. This is a relative term, and you still have to figure out total carbs by using your portion size, not the one on the bag, box or sticker!

Keto friendly: Suggests but does not guarantee you will not get bumped out of ketosis by consuming these foods – this category is extremely vague and variable, so you have to experiment on yourself.

Net Carbs: Frankly, this could be viewed as a deceptive marketing term. Low net carb containing foods often behave just like high carb foods – by spiking our appetites for sweets.

Again, it is recommended to avoid some foods from these categories, or at least be aware of the potential for a high-carb effect if you do consume them. Be especially cautious of "low net carb" meal replacement or "energy" bars, even if you see the word Keto on the label!

As you enter into ketosis, you will notice changes in how you feel.

First, there may be a feeling of "mental changes." Some people describe a mild elevation of mood or a mild fogginess that lasts just a few minutes. If you have ever been in and out of ketosis before, you already know if this happens to you.

Once you have attained and maintained ketosis, you will most likely notice you are passing more urine than usual. This accounts for some "water weight" loss that Keto diets are so famous for.

As we shall see later, the using up of stored glycogen (a form of sugar) also causes sizeable water loss in most people.

Do not be alarmed at either of these things.

The first is actually a byproduct of something called *saluresis*. As the body converts to ketones as a major fuel instead of blood sugar, the kidneys start to get rid of salt. This causes rapid weight loss, but it can also lead to one of the side effects that are commonly misinterpreted by people who are in ketosis. That side effect is *postural hypotension* – a fancy name for light-headedness that occurs when you bend over and stand up.

Most people misinterpret this as "low blood sugar". All that is needed is a little extra salt, or even a salt tablet, to get rid of the lightheadedness if it happens.

Keep in mind, if you have high blood pressure, consuming extra salt may not be a good option. Also, keep in mind that most medical professionals will say salt is deadly, because they do not account for it being in the context of ketogenic diets.

what the doctor won't tell you!

Now is a good time to address some of the typical concerns of medical professionals. Keep in mind that, as with any profession, medicine and paramedical occupations like Nutritionists and Dieticians have a certain source for information that is agreed upon by the profession.

Without realizing it, many health care professionals have an inherent bias for, and against, things that depend mainly on who is saying it and whether it fits with their current belief systems.

Sometimes, as is the case with ketogenic diets, there is a strong bias against diet or lifestyle approaches. Even in the scientific literature, there is a large body of "evidence" that "proves" high fat diets cannot be good for you. Dr. Dave's medical school days taught that this kind of diet was deadly. And the teachings were under the normal assumptions made in the medical profession. The accumulating evidence for the benefits of Keto diet, and the progression in our understanding of how to apply it, is changing these notions.

The main reasons why people may still feel these diets are unhealthy, and the fallacies behind those reasons, are as follows:

1) Ketogenic diets avoid carbs which are a major and necessary food group. This supposition is false for several reasons. First, carbs are not essential. Only fats and proteins are essential. Your body can easily make everything it needs from fats and proteins. Carbs are non-essential nutrients, and you can live an entire healthy lifetime with very small amounts of them.

   Next, it is virtually impossible to avoid all carbs, nor should you try. You should simply shoot to keep your total daily carb intake under 50 grams/day for a week or two while you also calorie-restrict. If you decide not to calorie-restrict at some point, then you may venture with carbs as high as 100 grams/day, at least on occasion. The scale and the amount of fat you are carrying on your waist (waste!) line will clue you in very quickly if this is too many carbs for you.

   Then you can begin to count the grams intake more closely and reduce your carbs to a level at which you can maintain both your health and physique.

   A reasonably crafted ketogenic diet leaves room for a healthy dose of green and other vegetables, as long as these are generally low carb. As far as fruits, most can be consumed in the form of various berries. Strawberries, blueberries and raspberries are all reasonably low carb and can be consumed in single handful amounts without much worry. Lots of greens and a few handfuls of various types of berries will provide you with plenty of vitamins and minerals that you need.

2) Ketogenic diets may cause ketoacidosis. It is important to know the difference between ketosis and ketoacidosis. *Ketoacidosis* is indeed a dangerous condition that is usually associated only with severe diabetes (especially type 1, or advanced type 2) or certain forms of kidney disease. In this condition, there is a complete lack of insulin and a completely dysregulated production of ketones. The body is basically unable to use any fuel, such as glucose (sugar) or ketones, and these build up in the bloodstream. Since ketone bodies are acidic, when enough of them build up, they make the blood become acidic, and this is a very dangerous condition.

   If you have normal healthy kidneys and are not insulin dependent or poorly regulated with your blood sugar, you have virtually no chance of going into ketoacidosis.

Ketosis is a NORMAL BENIGN condition that is the amazing result of the human body's ability to adapt to different fuel sources, such as to restricted calories or starvation. When carbohydrates and/or calories are significantly limited or absent, the body switches over to using ketone bodies as a normal fuel source. In both – a calorie restricted and non-calorie restricted ketogenic diet – the body will use dietary AND stored fat as its main source of fuel. Thus, your body will lean out.

Additional terms you might come across: *Calorie Restriction* vs. *Ad Libitum* diets. If you read any of the scientific literature on Ketogenic Diet, especially if it's recently conducted, you will see these phrases. The unrestricted calorie eating (ad libitum) during Keto dieting will support the state of nutritional ketosis. Restricting the calories during Keto (calorie restriction) can further advance the state of ketosis.

When you go Keto, fat and ketosis combined should suppress your appetite if you have a "normal" metabolic response. The end result is that you may consume about the same amount, or even fewer, calories as characteristic for an average-day appetite.

A great way to get into ketosis quickly is to calorie restrict to 500 calories of Keto type foods for 3 days. Most people will automatically be well into ketosis this way. It is theoretically possible to eat ad libitum (as much as you like) and get into keto state, but it has not proven to be achieved easily in our testing. The recommended approach to get into ketosis is by watching calories overall and reducing them by at least 20% of your typical intake (or more, if possible). Again, lowering the calorie intakes will make getting into keto state easier, and ultimately you will see faster fat loss.

3) Scientific studies on high fat diets often show an increase in inflammation in the body and an increase in cholesterol, with conclusions that these diets contribute to heart diseases. Universally the scientific studies on high fat diets have one or more of the following flaws:
   A) They are not truly high fat, and they still maintain a high portion of carbohydrates (carbs). The typical scientific study in high fat diets uses between 35% and 55% fat with the bulk of the rest of the diet being carbs followed by lower proteins. This is not a high fat diet. A high fat diet is between 60% and 70% of all calories consumed as fat and 15 to 20% as protein with a maximum of 10% carbs. We are not aware of any study that – with the use of the mentioned parameters – would arrive to negative conclusions of ketogenic diet effects when the studies are carried out for more than 10 days. There are many published studies in reputable journals that conclude that high fat diets are dangerous, however they tend to use carbs as a major, or simply too high a percentage, of the dietary calories. All this would do is show that high carb diets are dangerous!
   B) The studies are usually short duration. It is amazing how many studies have been done with a single high fat meal as the 'smoking gun' for this diet. The human body does not adapt to anything instantaneously except perhaps oxygen content and carbon dioxide! Yet, a single high fat meal (again, usually in the presence of high carbs as well) is "proof" that these diets are bad for you. This is an utter fallacy. If one allows a 2-week adaptation, all of the bad blood parameters begin to reverse and eventually exceed the expectation of the most demanding health care professionals. This is also in the literature, but few doctors and other health care professionals account for this information. You may have the best cholesterol values in your life eating a very high fat diet – so long as you avoid carbohydrates.
   C) They are sponsored by people who have a vested interest in proving that high fat is bad for you. This includes many pharmaceutical manufacturers who would have the entire population on statin drugs.

4) You cannot get good nutrition if all you eat is fatty meats. There is indeed some merit to this, although you might be surprised how good your blood numbers look if you maintain a long-term ketogenic diet. One thing to highly recommend is consuming only *grass-fed meats*.

Do not neglect this – all meat should be grass-fed free range whenever possible, not fed on grains. Smoked and cured meats are to be limited as well. Do not, however, be afraid of fattier cuts of meat. These meats, if grass fed, are loaded with the very healthy Omega 3 fats that you need.

Similarly, line caught or ocean caught non-farmed fish are essential.

As for dairy, raw is better, which, at least in most of the USA, means you must visit a farm to get this, as it is not usually allowed to be sold in retail stores. If you consume meats and dairy from these sources, the fats you get will be a perfect blend of what your body needs to remain a lean and healthy temple!

Explore the carb content of vegetables and fruits, and you will see that even on relatively severe restriction you will be able to consume a good amount of green leafy vegetables and several fruits, albeit in smaller quantities, than you might normally consume. A high-quality fish oil and a good multivitamin can easily make up any perceived deficits you might think you have.

5) You will only lose water weight on Keto diets. This, of course, is not true, because anyone taking diuretics (water pills) would get a 6-pack abdomen. What does happen early in keto diets is you DO use glycogen which is stored in a "hydrated" form (meaning water is associated with it). This weight does come off first and accounts for the oft seen couple of pounds a day weight loss early in your Keto diet. Losing weight does not last, but it is not uncommon to lose 5-7 pounds in the first week of Keto dieting. This will be accounted for, somewhat, by the obligate water that is "stored" with glycogen. But, soon after, the fat will also begin to melt away and the changes in your physique will convince you that it's not just water weight!

6) Once you go off this diet, you will gain all the weight back!

Maintaining a ketogenic diet forever is not that easy, although, the longer you stay on it the easier it is.

By reviewing the effects of ketogenic diet, with the accumulating evidence of how it works in the body, it becomes obvious with every diligently designed study that the diet effects are a natural and healthy way to eat.

Our willingness to gain the insight into how the human body and the appetite work, and how eating certain foods influences the body, offers us the opportunity to have food serve our wellbeing instead of enslaving our existence!

You should know, however, that when it comes to choosing to practice a diet, to truly see the expected effects, it is important to stay true to following the diet. There is no middle of the road here. Think of an American driving on one side of the road and trying to drive that way in the UK. The result is disastrous.

That is exactly why the traditional Western diet that many people eat is, in truth, deadly and dangerous. It contains large amounts of man-made fats coupled with large amounts of sugar and carbohydrates. This is true even if you follow the dietary recommendations of most of the American "expert panels". They recommend that 60%+ of calories per meal come from carbohydrates. This would mean that every single day you would consume in excess nearly 300 grams of carbohydrates a day.

The way this is disguised as "healthy" is what could be called "The Whole Grain Agenda." That agenda centers around grains and other sources of carbs to a degree that is in excess of what we are designed by Mother Nature to eat. This huge excess forms the basis for most dietary recommendations your doctor and other health care professionals will adhere to, and expect you to adhere to, as well.

Simply put, everything we have read and researched to date, leads to stating that high carb diets are the enemy of good health and long life.

But once again, be advised there is no middle ground here.

There is a very definite level of carbohydrate consumption that will cause YOU PERSONALLY to gain weight and fat. The same level will adversely affect your cholesterol and other important biomarkers in your body. Finding that level of carbohydrate intake is an individual task. You may not need to adhere to a ketogenic diet with 50 grams of carbs a day forever, but it's a really good place to start and maintain for at least a few months. You will amaze yourself with what you can achieve in both the looks and health department.

carbohydrate poisoning and tips and pitfalls experienced by ketogenic dieters

Among the most common experiences mentioned by ketogenic dieters, the following can be listed:

1) Sugar is addictive! If you don't think so, you will have an opportunity to explore this during the first 3 to 5 days of your ketogenic diet. During this time, it is highly recommended to bite the bullet and either water-fast for 1-3 days, or reduce your calories dramatically to 500 or less for 7 to 14 days. The easiest way to do this is to eat very limited quantities of high fat meat or dairy (for example, use heavy cream in small amounts; use bouillon or bone broth derived from soup bones or marrow bones, and of course generous quantities of green leafy vegetables).

2) Once you have conquered the first few days and gotten firmly into ketosis, your appetite will become much easier to manage and will cease to be a problem. What you will notice is just how habitual eating is. You may still get hungry around the times you normally eat, but a large glass of warm water with lemon juice for flavoring and some broth will eliminate the hunger rapidly!

3) One of the most amazing things you will notice is the change in your appetite, if you are a night-time eater!

From Dr. Dave's personal experience:

I used to always need something to eat at night before bed, which is one of the worst times to eat. Often, I would notice that once I started eating I didn't stop and wound up consuming several hundred to almost a thousand calories before bed time. Then, in the morning, 7 or 8 hours later, I would wake up ravenous again.

When I went Keto, I still would have these cravings on occasion, but if I did not succumb and "went to bed hungry," I would wake up not hungry. This amazed me because how could I be hungry and then wake up 8 hours later not ravenous!

Not only was I not ravenous, but I was able to develop a habit that serves me well to this day. I would sleep 7 to 8 hours (usually better since I had not eaten!) and then wait another 4 hours or more before I was hungry again.

In addition, fasting of any length of time got much easier!

This showed me how powerful habit and anticipation are in "appetite". If you are hungry just a few hours after you eat, chances are you ate some carbs that you should have avoided, and these are making you hungry. If you wait a bit when you get hunger signals, they will often disappear for hours. If you have waited 15 or more hours to eat, especially breakfast, and you are hungry, that is probably real hunger, and you can eat.

The most impressive illustration of a 'fake' hunger I can think of goes back several years, when I had a habit of going out on weekends for a large gourmet meal as a celebration of family and friends. We would sit and eat and drink an enormous amount of calories over a 3-hour period. If and when alcohol was consumed, and dessert as well, the total calorie count could easily have been close to 2000 calories, with the carb count for that one meal exceeding 300 to 400 grams. It would take about an hour to get home from a favorite country inn, and I would be hungry again! Invariably, the next day I would over-eat as well before I could get control of my appetite.

Without going into a lot more detail, this represents the worst effects of what I call Carbohydrate Poisoning – my term for the regular consumption of excessive carbohydrates and the interaction with excess insulin, which causes rapid up- and down- turns of blood sugar, and in the long run many health consequences.

If you are familiar with the concept of a "cheat day," which is so prevalent in the body building literature, it never worked for me and, honestly, I have never seen it work well for anyone over the age of 28! The cheat day supposedly resets the hormone leptin and allows you to continue on a low-calorie cutting diet to reduce your body fat. I think the concept is flawed because it ignores a bigger more potent and fast-acting hormone called Insulin!

Our goal is to stay in ketosis for prolonged periods of time. Once you bounce out of ketosis, it will take you several days to get back in, as if you were starting from scratch. Why put yourself through that?

Why nullify the hard-won health and physique benefits you've earned by implementing the new eating habits.

Simply put: Once in ketosis, stay in ketosis for as long as it serves you! If you decide to come out of ketosis once you've spent a few months there, choose a lower carb variety of diet so you do not reverse the bulk of the benefits you just achieved. For most people, the way they look and feel is reward and incentive enough to stay on ketosis long-term.

4) Beware of high caffeine intakes. Without going into too much biochemistry, lowering the caffeine intake is important. Sometimes, this is a problem, because you are "giving up" sugar and caffeine, both of which are addictive. A practical rule-of-thumb advice is to reduce the daily caffeine consumption gradually – by a third, then by another third; or to limit your caffeine to 50 milligrams, or the equivalent of one strong cup of coffee a day. It is best to consume the beverage several hours before you eat your first meal. Implied in this is that you may wake up, consume some water and caffeine, and then wait until "lunch" to actually eat your first meal.

Perhaps the biggest oversight for Ketogenic Diet followers is consuming low, rather than sufficient, amount of fat in the diet! Rarely, consuming too much protein may become an issue, especially if it's taken in the later part of the day. Recent research suggests that protein over-consumption is rarer than originally thought.

People on the Carnivore Diet – another version of Keto – have no such problems even though they eat a lot of meat. BUT, remember, this is a high fat diet! Cheeses, heavy cream, nuts and some meats (for example, uncured bacon for the fat, as well as fatty meat cuts) are the mainstay of the Keto diet choices.

5) The great leveler for anticipated results from Keto diet is in regulating calories.

From Dr. Dave's personal experience:

When I first went onto a low-calorie ketogenic induction, I used a product called Ideal Protein. This company makes many extremely low carb but relatively high protein products. Because I limited my calorie intake to 300 to 400 calories a day, even the high protein per serving of 20 grams (total 60 grams a day) was not enough to bump me out of ketosis. Although, getting into ketosis did take a lot longer (3 days to begin to get into real ketosis) than when water-fasting (which took less than 48 hours to get to 1.0 mmol/L (0.6 mmol/L UK).

6) READ THIS CAREFULLY PLEASE: There is a small subset of people who have a derangement that is caused by defects in how they handle appetite. No one has quite figured out the pathway, but the problem seems to be in the brain itself. By far, the bulk of people will enjoy a significant reduction in hunger/appetite when consuming a high fat diet. This includes people who claim to be born to be obese, have the thrifty gene, etc. The trick for most people is to get through the first 3 to 5 days of calorie restriction and allow the appetite squashing effects of ketosis to prevail. Then your body becomes a fat burning machine, your inflammatory biochemistry reverts to a non-inflamed state, your health improves, your body takes out the trash, and maintaining the diet becomes easy.

7) One of the most common excuses of not wanting to try a ketogenic diet for health, wellness, or weight loss reasons is: "I can't give up MY BREAD" (or pasta)." This is pure cultural nonsense! If you really honestly believe you cannot limit or give up bread, then find someone who has taken on the challenge and ask them to share their results. Their success will inspire you to have a serious look at what you are – a human being first, capable of accomplishing what you set your mind to. You were born human, you merely inherited your culture!

What is a high fat diet? This is so important it is worth reiterating: High fat refers to consuming 65 to 70 % of your calories from fat, and the rest – ~20% from protein and ~10% or less from carbs.

As mentioned earlier, most studies on high fat diets fall far short of these numbers and are in fact High Carb diets with more than usual fat in them. The sequela are deadly and this is exactly what the studies show without meaning to: consume a lot of carbs with relatively more fat than usual, and disease and death rates go up in the laboratory subjects in the studies.

Every one of these studies had around 35% fat, meaning the rest was Carbs and protein! Let's say that the protein intake was 25% of the calories. You now have 60% of 100% of calories from non-carb sources and a whopping 40% from Carbs. Thus, these studies were done with High Carb Diets, not High Fat Diets!

Carbs kill! Not fats.

keto flu and what to do!

In the first 3 to 4 days of Keto diet, people may experience a low energy state, or "keto flu." It is more likely to occur when you are calorie restricting. This state is temporary and can be accompanied by lightheadedness and a "funny feeling" of disconnectedness.

During this time, a little bit of salt and some water will go a long way with rebalancing the body. Reducing your workout load by up to 50% will help with rebalancing the mind. Have no fear, this doesn't last, and you'll love the way and the speed at which your body changes once in ketosis.

Finally, if you can actually fast 24 hours at a time for a few days with just one reasonably sized Keto meal, you will see remarkable changes and learn the key to controlling your eating habits – they are just that, HABITS! You will observe the moments of getting "hungry" at the usual times when you normally would eat. After 3 to 4 days, your hunger disappears, even though you did not eat.

Another amazing thing is you may "go to bed hungry" and wake up not wanting food at all. This shows you how much your eating is habitual.

Resist these typical eating times for just a few days (it's quite hard!), and you will be cured of "Habitual Hunger." Similarly, if you choose to exercise and get hungry after you work out, the urge to eat will usually pass after 30 minutes.

Committing to the first 3 to 4 days while transitioning to Keto diet is likely to re-open the alertness, resilience and clarity in your body and mind like you remembered from the days of high school!

epigenetics and keto – the key to all good things for most of us!!

Epigenetics is all the rage these days and is often used and misused to support various diets, which at times make no sense from an evolutionary standpoint.

Epigenetics literally means around or near the genome. The Genome is the vast array of DNA material we have that codes for cells and tissues that make us who we are. DNA material is what we pass on to our children. DNA is very much the blueprint of who we are physically, and in some cases mentally.

DNA also contains signals that regulate and time the events inside individual cells as well as other cells both near and far in the body. The body has trillions of cells and most of them carry some sort of DNA genetic material.

The DNA genetic material is arranged in its own spiral fashion called a "double helix" that winds around itself like a spiral staircase. But, in fact, that description, which is the one most of us are first exposed to in Biology Class, is oversimplified.

DNA is actually much more tightly coiled most of the time and covered by specific proteins. A common type of protein found mixed in or immediately around the DNA is called a histone. Histones are subject to modification and change that, in turn, allows or denies access to the DNA for the purpose of "making or not making things from the blueprint."

In short, epigenetics controls which genes are read and not read and which genes influence or do not influence us. This is why the mere presence of an unhealthy gene or healthy gene is not a death sentence or a free pass to do what you want in your lifestyle!

The epigenome, that group of proteins that controls which genes are turned on or off, can also be inherited. Children are born with many of the epigenetic "marks" or histone modifications of their mother (the mother's influence seems to be greater in epigenetics!). The main difference between the genome (DNA) and the epigenome is that it may take thousands or millions of years for a gene that is useful to become stably integrated into the human genome.

Contrary to the changes in genome speed, your epigenome can change in seconds, minutes, hours, days or weeks.

Another way to look at the definition of the epigenome and Epigenetics is "Where the environment meets the genome." This is where our lifestyle choices, including, of course, what we eat, has a huge influence on our health.

The contemporary Western Diet has massive effects on our epigenome. Most of the effects are not supportive of our body's strength and resilience, and this is one of the reasons why we suffer so much as a species, especially as we get older.

The ketogenic diet has MASSIVE and healthy influences on the epigenome. Indeed, that is where most of the health benefits come from – in the switching on and off of genes that are healthy or unhealthy for us in the context of what we eat. If you think back to our "ancestral you and me," the ketogenic diet fits perfectly with what we were "designed" to eat. It is our natural diet.

food groups – putting keto in context

It may seem strange to introduce the topic of Food Groups this late in the text. We are about to get into the Recipes section. So by introducing the Food Groups, now you will be able to see specifically where each food group is featured or omitted. You will clearly see the low carb aspect of these recipes!

There are 3 main food groups or "macro" food groups if you will: carbohydrates, proteins, and fats.

Each of them has a very different biochemical makeup or signature form that defines them.

The chemical structure of *carbohydrates* consists of carbon, hydrogen, and oxygen atoms, usually with a ratio of 2 to 1 hydrogen to oxygen. This food group includes sugars, starches and fibers. The main source of this food group is grain based in the modern Western Diet. While it is true that fiber is often "low in sugar," most of the foods in the carbohydrate group cause insulin secretion and are easily and commonly converted to sugar by the human body.

Wherever sugar happens in the body, insulin also happens (with the exception of type 1 diabetes and some other very rare endocrine conditions). Remember insulin is the fat storage hormone. No other food group has the capacity to stimulate insulin to the same degree as carbohydrates, so no other food group has the capacity to make us as fat as carbohydrates can.

But if you are like many people, the thought of avoiding all carbs is scary to you. Not to worry – it is almost impossible to avoid all carbs. If you buy and eat anything in a can or a package, you are getting some carbs. If you eat as you should, vegetables and a little fruit daily, you are getting carbs. So do not worry, you will almost always have a daily intake of some carbs!

On a per gram basis, pure carbohydrates contain 5 calories.

On a ketogenic diet, most people will need to keep their carbohydrate intake below 50 grams daily. If they exceed that, the carb content will stimulate insulin to the degree that it inhibits ketosis, and the body will switch back to using carbs as a primary food source.

Another way to look at the day's intake of carbs is by total calorie intake: carbs should not exceed 5 to 10% of your total calorie intake on a daily basis.

Now let us talk about *proteins*.

There are 21 amino acids that make up proteins. Nine of them are essential, meaning YOU MUST get them from the diet.

In addition to containing carbon, hydrogen, and oxygen atoms, proteins also contain nitrogen, and often sulfur and phosphorus. Proteins are essential for connective tissue and muscle. As individual molecules, they make up many of the structures and signaling molecules of the cell. Proteins do stimulate insulin, sometimes as much as carbohydrates do. This is primarily to assure that muscle takes up the protein it needs. It was mentioned earlier that insulin is THE FAT STORAGE hormone. This is true, but it is a simplification. Insulin is, in more general terms, a "growth" hormone. One of its actions is to stimulate muscle growth.

While protein does stimulate insulin, protein does not spike the blood sugar the way carbs do. Nor does it provide the easy source of calories that most carbs, especially grain based or added sugar foods, do. Protein has a very high "thermic" effect (calories used to digest it). Simply put, this means your body has to work very hard to get at the calories that protein provides.

On a per gram basis, pure protein provides only 4 calories, making it the lowest calorie source in the diet.

Too much protein can also bump you out of ketosis though! This is because protein can be used to create sugar, especially at night while we sleep, by a process called Gluconeogenesis. Literally, this means "the making of new glucose," with protein being the primary source for the process. This is one reason why we do not suffer from excessively low blood sugars while we sleep. Protein is naturally broken down, or catabolized, while we sleep to provide enough sugar to keep the body running during the time we are not eating.

If this sugar production becomes excessive, it will also bump you out of ketosis, just like too many carbs will.

People on a ketogenic diet should limit their protein intake to 15 to 20% of their total calories. For most women, this is below 30 grams of protein daily, and for most men – below 85 grams per day.

Remember, the ketogenic diet changes EVERYTHING about the way your body uses macro food groups. Even if you exercise hard and do a lot of weight training or running, you do not need to increase the protein intake by more than 10% of the above numbers! Doing so will bump you out of ketosis and defeat the purpose and health benefits of this diet!

Now let us talk about *fats*.

Fat molecules contain primarily carbon and hydrogen atoms and are the most efficient form to store energy.

Fat is the basis of the ketogenic diet because when fat is used as the main fuel for the body, ketones are produced as the major fuel for both the body and the brain.

While the brain still uses sugar, as does the rest of the body, it does not require the major amounts that you would have to provide if you were eating carbs. Sugar becomes more of a background fuel, and ketone bodies – primarily Beta-hydroxybutyrate (BHB) – become the main fuel source.

From Dr. Dave's clinical experience:

One of the common criticisms I get, when I "recommend" a high fat diet, goes like this (and usually comes from a nutritionist or dietician): "I am not about to eliminate or limit one of the major essential food groups that has heretofore made up the bulk of my calories. It MUST be unhealthy to focus on one kind of food group to the exclusion of all others! Therefore, this high fat ketogenic diet you speak of cannot be healthy for me or anyone else!"

In point of fact, as mentioned before, carbs are NOT ESSENTIAL for survival!

I have personally experienced blood sugars in the 30's while maintaining nutritional ketosis (3.0 to 4.0 mmol/L) with no issues in functioning whatsoever.

There are 2 essential fats (fatty acids) known for humans: An Omega 6 fat, called Linoleic Acid, serves as a building block for many of the inflammatory chemicals in our body, as well as many cell membrane structures; and the Omega 3 fat Linolenic Acid, which is the building block for anti-inflammatory compounds and cell membranes as well.

From Dr. Dave's clinical observations:

> *Many people consider the marine fatty acids EPA and DHA as the essential Omega 3 fats for humans because the primarily plant based Linolenic Acid is poorly converted to EPA and DHA. This is why many vegetarians and vegans have extremely low EPA and DHA levels!*
>
> *For the record, note the spelling difference between parent Linoleic Omega 6 and parent Linolenic Omega 3. Unlike the "parent" Omega 3's, Omega 6 is easily converted, outcompetes the Omega 3's in the conversion pathway and is present in EXCESS amounts in the Western Diet.*
>
> ***I recommend supplementing with Omega 3's, specifically fish oil, no matter what diet you maintain!***

The bottom line is: You can theoretically live without carbs, because THERE ARE NO ESSENTIAL CARBOHYDRATES! You cannot go very long without proteins or fats, without starting to show signs of disease, deterioration and eventually death. With this being said, eliminating carbs completely, even with the Ketogenic diet, is neither possible, nor practical. Regulating low carb intake is key.

ketosis and longevity – an emerging secret!

Because Ketosis naturally leads to appetite suppression and calorie restriction at least of a sort, it is common and very easy for people to link it with the practice of Intermittent Fasting.

Intermittent Fasting generally translates into longer times between the last meal of one day and the first meal of the next, e.g. supper to breakfast interval. Dr. Dave's recommendation of an interval for fasting is a minimum of 14-16 hours. This leaves about an 8-hour window for your meals. Generally, this results in the first meal being a bit bigger, since you haven't eaten, and the second being a bit smaller because you ate 6-8 hours ago.

It also makes "one meal a day" eating feasible and easy.

The effect of prolonged fasting facilitates *Cellular Recycling*, which includes the fostering of a very important process in your body called *Apoptosis*.

This literally means "controlled programmed cell death" and is part of the body's healthy normal recycling process. It is linked to another process that begins with the letter "A," *Autophagy*, which means "self-eating."

Self-eating leads to an orderly recycling of essential cellular components and gets rid of damaged ones that may be impairing critical cell processes and your overall health.

More importantly, these processes have been studied in both long-lived animals and longest-lived humans and are better and more efficient in the longest-lived of each. It seems apparent that Cellular Recycling is a critical step to making life at least as long as it "should" be!

An oft cited example of how long and well we "should live" is Jean Calmet.

She died at 122 years and was the world's oldest documented human. She rode a bike until 110, smoked and drank in moderation until 117.

More radical life extension will take adding telomerase activation and stem cells, but getting to the pre-programmed maximum life span in healthy fashion, with the Keto diet potentially facilitating it, is the first step! And the Keto approach is available to anyone.

So now that we know that efficient cellular recycling is essential to reach longer healthier life spans, we need to know one other huge process that is attached to ketosis with Intermittent Fasting.

This process is called *Amino Acid Recycling*.

Amino Acids are the building blocks for proteins in our body. As mentioned earlier, there is a total of 21 of them. Nine of these are essential, meaning they MUST be obtained through the diet – they cannot be made from others the way the non-essential amino acids can.

While the essential amino acids are super critical for health, it is the non-essential amino acid cysteine (made by oxidizing the non-essential amino acid cystine) that is the most important one in longevity, barring deficiencies of others.

Cysteine contains sulfur and is the building block for the body's most important antioxidant Glutathione. Drops in cysteine level can lead to drops in glutathione, which, in turn, lead to increased free radical facilitated oxidation, stress, and damage.

Another phenomenon related to protein metabolism and epigenetics is the production of peptides that favor repair, growth and physical characteristics associated with looking, feeling and being metabolically younger. (Of note, peptides are currently the new rage in Anti-Aging and Regenerative Medicine, so expect to hear a lot more about them in the near future.)

Aging is a disease of increasing low grade inflammation and free radical damage that cannot be repaired. Maintaining cysteine and glutathione levels counters both these aging effects directly and indirectly and, like efficient apoptosis and autophagy, has been shown to extend life and health spans.

So, now we have 2 direct reasons – Cellular Recycling and Amino Acid Recycling (and one indirect in Peptide metabolism), – which start addressing why Ketogenic Diets may extend both life and health spans.

There is another reason to mention – lowering insulin levels.

Most people are aware that insulin is related to blood sugar, and blood sugar is related to diabetes. Most people are also aware that these conditions are damaging to health. Eating a low carb diet automatically lowers insulin secretion and restores sensitivity to insulin that is often lost on our high carb diets. Catch these issues early enough, and you can reverse type 2 diabetes – the most common form in our adult population.

Everything mentioned in the above few paragraphs involves a key metabolic pathway called mTOR. Its regulation can lead to better mitochondrial health (the powerhouses of the cell), less inflammation, lower insulin levels and relatively higher antioxidant levels in the body. All of this is key in "anti-aging" your body!

Most people do not know that excess insulin secretion directly and indirectly affects the processes of apoptosis and autophagy in negative fashion: high insulin levels reverse the life extension benefits of these processes. Fortunately, they are easy to restore with Ketogenic Diets.

Finally, a word on Cancer and Calorie Restricted Diets. Our friend Dr. Thomas Seyfried recommends treating cancer with a combination of calorie restriction and ketosis. He has shown and summarized some remarkable case studies in his book "Cancer as a Metabolic Disease." This is a recommended reading for all health care professionals.

His hypothesis – that cancer starts with a respiratory defect in the mitochondria – has been echoed since the Nobel Prize was awarded to Otto Warburg in 1931. It is beyond the scope of this book to delve further into this hypothesis, but it was one of the driving forces that led us into exploring the Keto diet which now (2020) is the Keto craze!

Once you are Keto, you should stay Keto for as long as possible as the benefits accrue with time!

The influences of Ketogenic Diet mentioned in this chapter, in a very simple and not-too-scientific nutshell, are the reasons Ketogenic Diets should be viewed as Longevity and Life Extension Diets.

CHAPTER 10

I do THIS all the time!

By David M. Woynarowski, M.D.:

I'd like to share an email with you that was sent out to my specific readership on www.thelongevityedge. com. I am leaving it in the unedited format, just as it was the day I sent it. If you like being informed and updated on the topic of extended Health Span (how much of your life is spent in great health) and Life Span, go to the site and sign up for my emails!

In addition to practicing the Keto diet all the time, I also write emails regularly about Longevity topics.

****

"Ketone Drinks and Longevity"

You may realize if you've read some of my stuff anytime in the past 18 years that I have one major driving mission in life – to extend health span and, whenever possible, extend healthy life span.

Today's installment is not exactly new. I have written about this in the past 2-3 years on 2 other occasions, but today I am going to be a bit more 'sciencey' and a bit more blunt in terms of telling you what to do.

In reaching out to people who are "influencers" on social media, the discussion of keto diets brings a kind of 'on' or 'off' switch. I am finding most people are either for or against keto topic, based on very limited information. Most of that information centers around fat loss and aesthetics vs. the "unbalanced nature" of ketogenic diets.

One dietician wrote: "I don't see how you can recommend a diet that gets rid of one of the 3 essential food groups." She was of course referring to carbs. I didn't bother telling her that carbs are 1) Almost impossible to delete from the diet completely and 2) Not an essential food group. With simple supplementation like my Young Life Daily, you can skip carbs and your body will not fall into the Black Hole of nutritional deficiency or illness.

These concepts along with a lot of research are finally beginning to get into the brains of those who make nutrition a sole profession.

What I want to talk about today is the simple issue of longevity.

There exists in the body a complex metabolic regulator pathway known as mTOR, the mammalian target of Rapamycin – no I didn't invent the name. The name has nothing to do with its major function really. It is not solely based on the drug Rapamycin, although some are now selling routines using this as an anti-aging therapy. Viz a viz the topic of taking Rapamycin for life extension, I personally prefer using the keto diet instead of taking potentially immunosuppressant drugs, even in low doses.

This pathway, mTOR, leads to multiple effects, but when it is inhibited, at least in fruit flies and some lower mammals, it lengthens life. The mechanisms it works by are 3 Biggies (we'll skip some of the smaller ones for now!)

1) It (mTOR inhibition) helps your cells take out the cellular trash – degraded proteins, abnormally cross-linked proteins, lipofuscin granules (think pigments) and most of all gets rid of sick, dead, and dying mitochondria via a process called mitophagy. The net result of this is better power for your cells, and fewer toxic elements to inhibit metabolic functions and inflame the intracellular milieu. All of the negative effects mentioned can ultimately foster DNA damage. I just basically condensed a whole book into one paragraph but you get the message! Let me take this opportunity to recommend you remember your fish oil so you can increase the intracellular signals of healing: Resolvins and Protectins, both of which are derived from monoesters of Omega 3.

A footnote on Omega 3: Much has been made about the chemical format of Omega 3- ethyl ester, phospholipid, or triglyceride. The cell has any and all enzymes it needs naturally to use any format of Omega 3 you take. The only real difference is the speed of absorption of each format which becomes clinically meaningless when you consider the several-week time frame it takes for these fatty acids to equilibrate in your body. For reasons of purity, I prefer ethyl ester.

2) mTOR inhibition decreases the inflammatory and excessive growth effects of insulin signaling. Look at number 1) above for why this is important along with the potential to decrease our diabetes and obesity epidemics (all of which are related to excess carb intake!!!)

3) mTOR inhibition causes the transcription of hundreds of genes that decrease intracellular (and thus extracellular) inflammation including genes that code for superoxide dismutase, NFkB, catalase, glutathione peroxidase etc.

Now why is all this important?

Well, 2 reasons: Because you can mimic the effects of calorie restriction with ketone bodies, including those that you drink; and next, all of this decreases inflammation in your body.

The seminal role of Inflammation in Aging is described in a paper I co-authored below (*) and has since been expounded on greatly by others. The whole concept of "Inflammaging," which is now widely accepted, is based on inflammation as a cause of aging.

We also know that in "normal" people the expression of inflammatory genes increases as they age. This is due to epigenetic changes. As you might guess, this is also pointing to another favorite topic of mine – telomeres, but that is for another day!

References:

* Rafael Gonzalez, Dave Woynarowski, and Luis Geffner. Stem Cells Targeting Inflammation as Potential Anti-Aging Strategies and Therapies. Cell & Tissue Transplantation & Therapy. 2015, 7:1-8. Review.

Note: the following article offers scientific reasons why ketogenic diets and ketone drinks MAY be involved in longevity but does not guarantee any of same results for you. Educate yourself and see if the information stated makes sense, and then proceed as your own personal choices and health care professionals direct you!

Veech et al. Ketone Bodies Mimic the Life Span Extending Properties of Calorie Restriction. IUBMB Life. 2017, 69:305. Review.

****

Bottom line: My interest in Keto diet as a lifestyle is for the body's ability to use ketones as a major fuel instead of blood sugar. This switch carries a potential to advance Health Span and Life Span. Even when you use exogenous ketone drinks, like my Keto Gen, you will see normal blood sugars.

The reason I make a Keto Gen product and released this recipe book on the topic is not because it's in vogue or because you will look great on the diet (although that doesn't hurt!).

It's because these changes, literally and figuratively, can make you younger!!!

And that is what I have always been about!

Dr. Dave 2/20/2020   www.thelongevityedge.com

about keto edge recipes

By Oksana Zagorodna, Ph.D.:

It was my great pleasure to have collaborated with Dr. Woynarowski on researching the cutting edge of an extremely popular Keto diet.

After having researched cancer and metabolism in my graduate and postgraduate work, it was most exciting to team up with the esteemed medical professional and the Anti-Aging Medicine expert, to generate this book. Our project is an example of how scientific knowledge can be put to use in real time, through understanding the value of our food by learning the ingredients. With this knowledge, we can maintain and strengthen our health with smart nutrition, literally every day, one meal at a time.

Every recipe in this book has been meticulously thought through for the details of ingredients. In many recipes, the ingredients combined fortify each other's presence by boosting the absorption of the active ingredients to further support and strengthen our body.

You will find that, throughout the recipes, the nutrition content was kept high, the carbohydrate content was kept low. Each meal has a Keto Edge featured ingredient, which is mentioned with scientific evidence for its known active compounds and their effects in the body.

The ingredients that often involve spices create delicious combinations. Some of these ingredients have been used, for hundreds of years, for their taste; some were thought to benefit human body; and some have been applied to treat various ailments. But the scientific reasons behind their successful use were rarely available.

The difference now is that we can use the already accumulated and growing scientific knowledge to further tune our diet and to make every meal on our table nutritionally smarter.

Disease prevention starts at home.

Wellness does not have to vanish or fade with age. Having studied metabolic pathways in my cancer research work, I am amazed at how resilient and supportive our body is.

There should be no reason that we feel sluggish or tired after any given meal. And if we do, the food we ate was somehow unbalanced or unfitting for our body's health. We then have a choice – to continue eating as we did, or to change something for the better.

Small tweaks in our diet and habits can have the greatest effect and make a difference in the body beyond expected. For example, we are learning that limiting the hours of consuming food in a day to 6-8 hour windows is supportive for our health and wellness (if breakfast is at 10 am, the latest meal would be at 6 pm). The hours of eating can be as important as the ingredients that we use in every meal.

Making changes one meal at a time is an easy way to make a substantial difference in a lifestyle.

While the ingredients in every meal have their values individually, there is then an added value in how they come *together* to serve the body. For example, it is useful to know that raw broccoli is absorbed faster and in greater availability than cooked. Or that the benefits of turmeric are experienced at greater levels when consuming turmeric spice is coupled with black pepper.

Or, adding vanilla to a meal can make it seem sweeter. This creates an opportunity to decrease sugar use and intake. If we are on a healthy track with maintaining balanced nutrition and lifestyle, the reward is the sweetest – health, energy, and vitality.

Below is a summarized list of the ingredients that are featured throughout the Keto recipes in this book. With Keto being a high-fat diet, these ingredients can be added to the high-fat food sources such as beef, pork, chicken, and dairy, or vegetarian source of high fat such as avocado. These ingredients will improve the taste, the nutritional value, and the health benefits of any given recipe. You will find additional information on each of these ingredients in their respective featured recipe chapters.

Keto Edge Ingredients:

ALLSPICE (in "Meat & Fish") – contains molecules that are researched for reducing inflammation, regulating cardiovascular health, and showing antitumor effects.

ALMOND (in "Soups") – almond skin flavonoids (ASL) were shown to protect cholesterol in the body from oxidation.

AVOCADO (in "Meat & Fish") – contains numerous nutrients, vitamins, and phytochemicals; researched for chemoprevention purposes.

BEETS (in "Soups") – phytochemical molecules in beets have been studied in lab to lessen tumor cell growth through various mechanisms, including the inhibition of pro-inflammatory enzymes and the inhibition of lipid oxidation.

BLACK CURRANT (in "Desserts") – contains compounds that boost immunity, regulate blood pressure, exhibit antiviral and antibacterial properties, antioxidant and antiproliferative properties.

BLACK PEPPER (in "Meat & Fish") – supports digestion, regulates blood pressure and cholesterol levels; contains active compounds with antioxidant, anticancer and anti-inflammatory properties.

BROCCOLI (in "Breakfast") – contains a compound sulforaphane that has been shown to reduce cancer development and recurrence, and is well utilized in chemoprevention studies. Sulforaphane is an antioxidant and can activate the detoxifying enzymes in the body. It was shown to ameliorate obesity and insulin resistance in mice.

BRUSSELS SPROUTS (in "Sides") – contain molecules that can provide digestive support, detox support, regulate inflammation, boost immunity, researched for protecting against cancer.

CACAO POWDER (in "Desserts") – contains flavanols with potent antioxidant and anti-inflammatory effects; researched for anticancer properties.

CARDAMOM POWDER (in "Desserts") – contains compounds that help with regulating digestion, inflammation, oral health, exhibits antimicrobial properties and is studied in lab for anticancer effects.

CAULIFLOWER (in "Sides") – contains nutrients that boost and regulate digestive health, heart health, inflammation related conditions, researched for cancer-preventive effects.

CILANTRO (in "Breakfast") – studied for the antifungal, anti-inflammatory, antioxidant properties; the extract of Coriandrum Sativum was found to have reduced skin photoaging.

CINNAMON, GROUND (in "Desserts") – loaded with antioxidants, shows anti-inflammatory properties, may reduce the risk for heart disease, can reduce insulin resistance, lower blood sugar, treat infections.

CLOVES (in "Meat & Fish") – contains compounds that are used for the antiseptic and antiviral properties; researched for potential anticancer effects.

COCONUT CREAM (in "Sides") – contains nutrients that regulate weight, cardiovascular and neurological health.

CORIANDER (in "Salads") – contains beneficial antioxidants that can protect from diseases and boost the immune system.

CRANBERRIES (in "Desserts") – known to be used in treating urinary tract infections, boost immunity, boost circulation, reduce cardiovascular disease, support gut health.

CUMIN (in "Soups") – contains active compounds known to show gastroprotective, antioxidative, and neuroprotective effects.

DILL (in "Sides") – contains antioxidants that may help with lowering blood sugar, detoxifying foreign compounds in the body.

EGGPLANT (in "Salads") – contains molecules that can powerfully scavenge free radicals and have protective activity against lipid degradation in cell membranes (peroxidation).

GARLIC (in "Sides") – antimicrobial, immune booster, regulates cholesterol and blood pressure, circulatory stimulant, helps fight parasites and has cancer-fighting effects.

GINGER POWDER (in "Breakfast") –known to assist with a variety of powerful therapeutic and preventive effects used for thousands of years, to treat various symptoms from colds to cancer.

HORSERADISH (in "Salads") – contains phytochemicals studied for cancer-preventive properties.

LEMON ZEST (in "Breakfast") – contains terpenes, has well-established chemopreventive activity against various cancers.

LIME JUICE (in "Meat & Fish") – contains flavonoids with antioxidant abilities, found to assist with combatting cancers.

LIVER (in "Meat & Fish") – contains compounds that are important for brain development, nervous system functions at large, normal metabolism and transport of lipids.

NUTMEG (in "Salads") – studied for preventing cancer.

ONIONS (in "Sides") –contain quercetin, a flavonoid helpful in eliminating free radicals in the body.

PAPRIKA (in "Meat & Fish") – contains active compounds thought to regulate vision, cholesterol levels, inflammation, has antioxidant and anticancer effects.

PARSLEY (in "Soups") – supports heart health, digestion, bone health; a flavonoid molecule found in parsley has been repeatedly shown to have strong anticancer properties.

PECANS (in "Desserts") – contain compounds with antioxidant and neuroprotective properties, can regulate cholesterol; researched for inhibiting cancer cell growth.

PUMPKIN (in "Desserts") – contains compounds with antioxidant properties, boosts immunity, improves eyesight, may benefit heart health and aid in preventing cancer.

PUMPKIN SEEDS (in "Salads") – fiber-associated lignans found in pumpkin seeds may play a valuable role in preventing and treating breast cancer.

RADICCHIO LEAVES (in "Sides") – contain compounds to aid with digestion and colon cleansing, antiparasitic effects, antioxidant, can assist with weight loss and regulating body metabolism.

RED CABBAGE (in "Salads") – contains flavonoid antioxidants that are linked to lowering blood pressure, maintaining gut health, and keeping inflammation in check.

ROSEMARY, GROUND (in "Meat & Fish") – contains compounds that can improve digestion, alleviate muscle pain, boost the immune and circulatory system, improve memory, promote hair growth.

SALMON (in "Breakfast") – contains carotenoids and Omega 3 for antioxidant and anti-inflammatory effects.

SAUERKRAUT (in "Meat & Fish") – improves digestion, supports immune system, contains flavonoids that have been studied for decreasing the risk of several cancers.

SESAME OIL (in "Soups") – its content has been studied for its anti-inflammatory effects, regulating blood pressure, and for its effects in reducing photo-damage in lab studies in skin cells.

TAMARIND (in "Salads") – contains phytochemicals studied in lab for their antioxidant effects and for the effects in suppressing cancer cell growth.

THYME (in "Meat & Fish") – contains flavonoids high in the antioxidant activity, studied for the anticancer effects, immunity boosting, and antimicrobial activities.

TURMERIC (in "Meat & Fish") – well studied for its antioxidant, anticancer effects; well known for its anti-inflammatory contributions.

TURNIP (in "Sides") – known to have antioxidant, antimicrobial, anticancer properties, aids with digestive tract, regulates weight and blood pressure.

VANILLA (in "Desserts") – compounds have antioxidant, antidepressant, and antitumor effects.

WALNUTS (in "Meat & Fish") – support digestion, regulate blood pressure and cholesterol levels; boost immunity, reduce inflammation, rich in Omega 3 essential fatty acid.

Please enjoy, utilize these ingredients into recipes, and modify to your liking. We hope you put to good use the scientific, practical, and informative food examples that have come together in The Keto Edge.

We encourage you not to limit yourself solely to the information in this book, but to make it a starting point in your Keto journey. Keep in mind that the information is going to expand, evolve and grow in its scope for many years to come!

Here is to your health!

RECIPES

recipes

Salads

Easter Salad
Red & Green Cabbage Cole Slaw Salad
Eggplant Salad
Tomato Cucumber Romaine Salad
Mixed Leaf Tomato Salad with Pumpkin Seeds and Mozzarella
Cucumber Pepper Salad
Tomato Cucumber Salad with Nutmeg

Breakfast

Lemon Zest Muffins
Avocado Smoked Salmon Omelet
Loaded Ground Beef Scrambled Eggs
Egg Salad Chicken Wraps
Italian Baked Eggs

Soups

Cilantro Lime Meatball Soup
Chicken or Beef Soup with Almonds
Chia Mushroom Soup
Beet Soup (Borsch)
Spinach & Tofu Soup

Meat & Fish

Beefy Cauliflower & Almond Stir-Fry
Curry Beef Meatballs
Liver Pancakes
Kielbasa and Sauerkraut
Chicken Sausage with Zucchini Stir-Fry
Ginger Coconut Chicken
Lemon Pepper Chicken Legs (or Tenders)

recipes

Meat & Fish ~ Continued

Beefy Broccoli & Walnut Stir-Fry
Steak with Creamy Vegetable Topping
Spiced Beef Tips
Salmon Patties with Avocado
Salmon with Cucumber Sauce

Sides

Eggplant Pancakes
Salt-Roasted Turnip with Tomato and Goat Cheese
Fried Cauliflower
Stir-Fried Mushroom & Broccoli with Coconut and Walnuts
Roasted Purple Cabbage
Sautéed Parsnip Mushrooms
Brussels Sprouts and Bacon
Radicchio Eggplant Ragout

Desserts

Rich Chocolate Almond Loaf
Pumpkin Pie
Checkerboard Cake
Buttercream Rum Cake
Cranberry Thins
Almond Pecan Cookies
Chocolate Truffles
Dr. Dave's Ice Cream

salads

Easter Salad

Red & Green Cabbage Cole Slaw Salad

Eggplant Salad

Tomato Cucumber Romaine Salad

Mixed Leaf Tomato Salad with Pumpkin Seeds and Mozzarella

Cucumber Pepper Salad

Tomato Cucumber Salad with Nutmeg

Easter Salad

Serves 2

Ingredients

8 oz kielbasa (regular or smoked),
        cut in cubes
4 stalks of celery, chopped
4 hardboiled eggs, cut in cubes
4 stalks green onions, chopped
4-6 radishes, sliced
12 oz goat cheese (or feta cheese),
        cut in cubes
8 oz butter, cut in cubes
1 oz fresh horseradish root,
        shredded thinly
Salt and pepper to taste

Preparation

1. In a mixing bowl, combine the pre-cut ingredients: kielbasa, celery, boiled eggs, green onions, radishes, cheese, and butter.
2. Add the shredded horseradish root and salt/pepper.
3. Mix well.
4. Serve chilled.

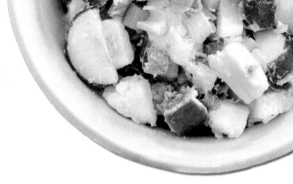

Enjoy!

Keto Edge featured ingredient: HORSERADISH

Among health-related properties/actions: Circulatory stimulant, decongestant, digestive, antimicrobial, expectorant, anthelmintic, anti-inflammatory, diuretic.

Among known active molecules/compounds: Glucosinolates – phytochemicals studied for cancer-preventive properties.

Sources:
J Agric Food Chem. 2015, 63(11):2947-2955.
https://pubs.acs.org/doi/abs/10.1021/jf505591z?journalCode=jafcau
Food Funct. 2015, 6(12):3778-88.
https://www.ncbi.nlm.nih.gov/pubmed/26411988
Prevent Disease May 19, 2016.
https://preventdisease.com/news/16/051916_Horseradish-Compounds-Which-Remove-Cancer.shtml
Prevent Disease March 13, 2014.
https://www.preventdisease.com/news/14/031314_Horseradish-More-Effective-Pharma-Clear-Sinus-Infections-Mucus-From-Respiratory-Passages.shtml

Red & Green Cabbage Cole Slaw Salad

Serves 4

Ingredients

1 cup thinly sliced green cabbage
1 cup thinly sliced red cabbage
½ cup chopped yellow or red bell pepper
¼ cup chopped red onion
2 oz goat cheese, crumbled
¼ cup mayonnaise
2 tbsp olive oil
Salt and pepper

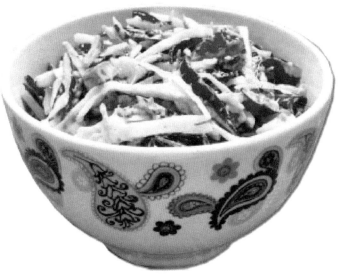

Preparation

1. Combine vegetables (green and red cabbage, bell pepper, red onion) and cheese in a bowl.
2. Add olive oil, mayonnaise, salt, pepper.
3. Mix and serve.

Enjoy!

Keto Edge featured ingredient: RED CABBAGE

Among health-related properties/actions: Antioxidant, anti-inflammatory, digestive, cardiovascular health, rich in nutrients (especially vitamins C, K).

Among known active molecules/compounds: Anthocyanins (including cyanidin) – flavonoid antioxidants that are linked to lowering blood pressure, maintaining gut health, and keeping inflammation in check.

Note: The greatest health benefits come from consuming raw cabbage.

Sources:
Food Chem. 2014, 145:77-85.
https://www.ncbi.nlm.nih.gov/pubmed/24128451
Am J Clin Nutr. 2012, 96(4):781-88.
https://www.ncbi.nlm.nih.gov/pubmed/22914551
ScienceDaily March 11, 2008.
www.sciencedaily.com/releases/2008/03/080307081409.htm

Eggplant Salad

Serves 2-4

Ingredients
1 large eggplant
½ cup water
1 onion
8 oz favorite salsa
Salt and pepper to taste
Garnish with dill or parsley

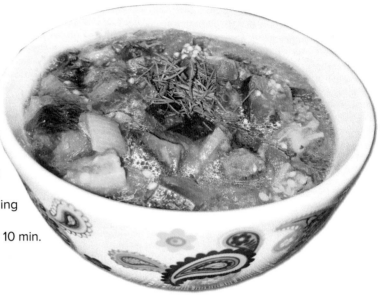

Preparation
1. In a large pot, bring water to a boil, add salt and pepper.
2. Cut the eggplant into cubes, add to the boiling water, and cook until soft (~10 min).
3. Add the salsa mixture and cook for another 10 min.
4. Serve warm or chilled. Garnish with dill.

Enjoy!

Keto Edge featured ingredient: EGGPLANT
Among health-related properties/actions: Antioxidant, anti-inflammatory, can assist with weight management, can prevent age-related vision loss, may help with preventing cancer cells from growing.

Among known active molecules/compounds: The well-recognized purple color of an eggplant skin is anthocyanin nasunin. Nasunin is a potent antioxidant that can powerfully scavenge free radicals and has protective activity against lipid degradation in cell membranes (peroxidation). Another antioxidant, a polyphenol, chlorogenic acid, was shown to improve blood cholesterol in rodents.

Sources:
Toxicol. 2000, 2-3:119-23.
https://pubmed.ncbi.nlm.nih.gov/10962130
Food Chem Toxicol. 2020, 135:110922.
https://www.ncbi.nlm.nih.gov/pubmed/31669599
Phytothera Res. 2012, 27(4):545-51.
https://onlinelibrary.wiley.com/doi/abs/10.1002/ptr.4751

Tomato Cucumber Romaine Salad

Serves 2

Ingredients

8-12 oz cucumbers (one big or two medium), chopped
8-12 oz tomatoes (red or yellow grape size tomatoes), chopped
2 medium radishes, chopped
2-4 oz romaine salad leaves (1 stem bunch), chopped
4 tbsp olive oil
1 tbsp mayonnaise
Salt, pepper, coriander to taste
Greens for garnishing (if desired)

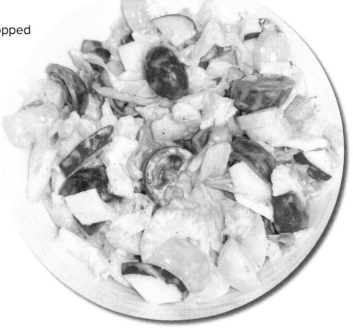

Preparation

1. In a mixing bowl, combine cucumbers and tomatoes (cut grape tomatoes in halves).
2. Add salt, pepper, coriander. Mix well.
3. Add radishes and romaine salad, mix in olive oil, mayonnaise.
4. Garnish with greens if desired.

Enjoy!

Keto Edge featured ingredient: CORIANDER

Among health-related properties/actions: Antibacterial, antioxidant, decongestant, digestive, anti-inflammatory, immune bosting, anticancer, neuroprotective effects.

Among known active molecules/compounds: A compound dodecenal was shown to have bacteria-fighting (antimicrobial) properties. A study of eight herbs found coriander (as well as basil) to contain the highest levels of beta-carotene, beta-cryptoxanthin, lutein, and zeaxanthin – all beneficial antioxidants that can protect from diseases and boost the immune system.

Sources:
Food Chem. 2015, 15(167):24-9.
https://www.ncbi.nlm.nih.gov/pubmed/25148954/
Plant Foods Hum Nutr. 2010, 65(2):164-9.
https://www.ncbi.nlm.nih.gov/pubmed/20443063
J Agric Food Chem. 2004, 52(11):3329-32.
https://www.ncbi.nlm.nih.gov/pubmed/15161192

Mixed Leaf Tomato Salad with Pumpkin Seeds and Mozzarella

Serves 4

Ingredients

7 oz mixed salad leaves
8 oz tomatoes of choice, chopped
4 oz mozzarella cheese, cut in small cubes
2 oz walnuts
1-2 oz pumpkin seeds
2 tbsp extra virgin olive oil
2 tsp balsamic vinegar
¼ tsp Himalayan salt
¼ tsp black pepper

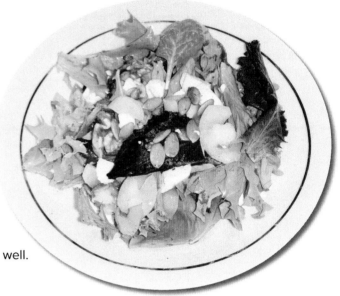

Preparation

1. In a large bowl, add the mixed salad leaves, tomatoes, mozzarella cheese, walnuts, and pumpkin seeds.
2. Add the oil and the vinegar, salt and pepper. Mix well.

Serve and enjoy!

Keto Edge featured ingredient: PUMPKIN SEEDS

Among health-related properties/actions: Antioxidants, anthelmintic, regulate blood pressure, regulate blood sugar, may help with preventing cancer.

Among known active molecules/compounds: Fiber-associated lignans found in pumpkin seeds may play valuable role in preventing and treating breast cancer; pumpkin seeds are a good source of magnesium which contributes to bone health (magnesium is often found deficient in adults).

Sources:
Nutr Cancer. 2013, 65(5):739-45.
  https://www.ncbi.nlm.nih.gov/pubmed/23859042
J Am Coll Nutr. 2009, 28(2):131-41.
  https://www.ncbi.nlm.nih.gov/pubmed/19828898
Food Res Internat. 2009, 42:641-46.
  https://doi.org/10.1016/j.foodres.2009.02.003

Cucumber Pepper Salad

Serves 2-4

Ingredients

1 cucumber (8 oz), thinly sliced into circles
¼ red bell pepper, thinly sliced into strips
2 tbsp lemon juice
½ tsp tamarind
2 tbsp black sesame oil
½ tsp sea salt
Garnish with cilantro
(If desired, soft cheese variety can be added)

Preparation

1. In a mixing bowl, combine the sliced cucumber,
    red bell pepper strips, lemon juice, tamarind, oil,
    and sea salt. Mix well.
2. Garnish with chopped cilantro.

Chill or serve instantly. Enjoy!

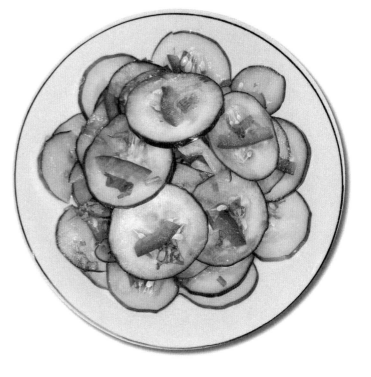

Keto Edge featured ingredient: TAMARIND

Among health-related properties/actions: Antioxidant, antimicrobial, anti-diabetic, regulates digestion, anti-inflammatory, anti-rheumatic, supports cardiovascular health.

Among known active molecules/compounds: When tested in lab, the phytochemical geraniol was shown to help with suppressing renal and pancreatic cell growth. Its therapeutic effects against cancer are thought to have important clinical and translational implications.

Sources:
Int J Oncol. 2016, 48(5):1772–82.
https://www.ncbi.nlm.nih.gov/pmc/articles/PMC4809657/
S Afr J Botany. 2010, 76:643-51.
https://www.sciencedirect.com/science/article/pii/S0254629910001559

Tomato Cucumber Salad with Nutmeg

Serves 2-4

Ingredients

1 cucumber (8 oz), chopped
2 medium size tomatoes, chopped
2 stalks of green onions, chopped
4 tbsp olive oil
½ tsp nutmeg
½ tsp sea salt
Garnish with cilantro
(If desired, soft cheese variety can be added)

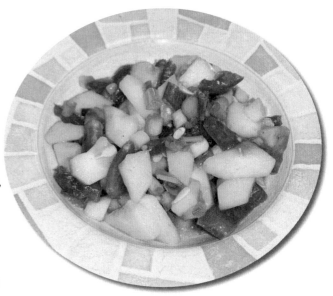

Preparation

1. In a mixing bowl, combine the chopped cucumber, tomatoes, nutmeg, and sea salt. Mix well.
2. Add the olive oil.
3. Garnish with chopped cilantro.

Chill or serve right away. Enjoy!

Keto Edge featured ingredient: NUTMEG

Among health-related properties/actions: Anti-inflammatory, antioxidant, antimicrobial, digestive, may enhance sex drive, circulatory stimulant, studied in preventing cancer.

Among known active molecules/compounds: Liquid fraction of Myristica Fragrans showed suppressed growth in cancer cells.

CAUTION: In large amounts, nutmeg can be toxic and create nausea and hallucinations.

Sources:
Am J Chin Med. 2016, 44:1063-79.
https://www.worldscientific.com/doi/abs/10.1142/S0192415X16500592
BMC Complement Altern Med. 2005, 5:16.
https://www.ncbi.nlm.nih.gov/pmc/articles/PMC1187868/
Phytochem Rev. 2016, 15(6):1035-56.
https://www.ncbi.nlm.nih.gov/pmc/articles/PMC5222521/

breakfast

Lemon Zest Muffins

Avocado Smoked Salmon Omelet

Loaded Ground Beef Scrambled Eggs

Egg Salad Chicken Wraps

Italian Baked Eggs

Lemon Zest Muffins

Serves 2-3

Ingredients
½ cup almond flour
¼ cup Truvia sweetener
½ teaspoon baking soda
4 eggs
¼ cup lemon juice
¼ cup coconut oil
Pinch of sea salt

Glaze:
3 tbsp heavy cream
½ tbsp Truvia sweetener
1 tsp lemon zest
Garnish with lemon zest and mint or basil leaves

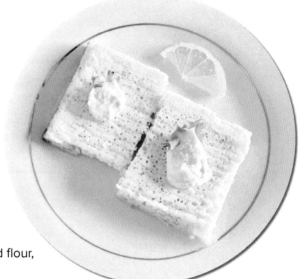

Preparation
1. Preheat the oven to 350°F.
2. In a medium-sized bowl, whisk together the almond flour, sweetener, and baking soda.
3. Add the eggs, coconut oil, lemon juice, and salt.
4. Distribute the batter on a muffin pan for muffins, or a rectangular baking sheet for bars. Bake for 10-12 min (check that the batter does not stick to the toothpick).
5. For the glaze:
   a. Mix heavy cream, sweetener, and lemon zest.
   b. Chill in the fridge (optional).
6. Remove the muffins from the oven and top each one with 1 tbsp of glaze, if desired.
7. Garnish with lemon zest and mint or basil leaves.

Eat warm. Best consumed when fresh. Enjoy!

Keto Edge featured ingredient: LEMON ZEST
Among health-related properties/actions: Antioxidant, antimicrobial, antifungal, cardiovascular, immune booster, may have anticancer properties.

Among known active molecules/compounds: A terpene found in lemon zest, D-limonene can aid with relief of heartburn and gastroesophageal reflux (GERD), and has been used clinically to dissolve gallstones. D-limonene has well-established chemopreventive activity against many types of cancer.

Sources:
Altern Med Rev. 2007, 12(3):259-64.
https://pubmed.ncbi.nlm.nih.gov/18072821-d-limonene-safety-and-clinical-applications/
Food Chem Toxicol. 2010, 48(1):99-106.
https://www.sciencedirect.com/science/article/pii/S027869150900430X?via%3Dihub
Phytomedicine. 2019, 53:37-42.
https://www.sciencedirect.com/science/article/abs/pii/S0944711318303088?via%3Dihub
Biomedicines. 2018, 6(2):70.
https://www.ncbi.nlm.nih.gov/pmc/articles/PMC6026940/

Avocado Smoked Salmon Omelet

Serves 2

Ingredients

1 tbsp lard or coconut oil
4 large eggs, beaten
2 tbsp heavy cream
2 oz smoked salmon, thinly sliced
¼ cup diced onion
2 tbsp Philadelphia cheese or goat cheese
¼ tsp ginger powder
1 medium avocado
Sea salt and pepper to taste
Greens for garnishing (dill, parsley)

Preparation

1. Whisk the eggs in a bowl; add heavy cream and mix; add salt, pepper, ginger powder.
2. In a pan, heat the oil (or lard).
3. Pour the egg over the mixture in the skillet. Cook over medium heat until the egg mixture starts solidifying. Once the mixture starts solidifying, divide it in the middle with the spatula, for 2 individual portions of the omelet.
4. Add 1 tbsp of cheese on each of the 2 omelet halves, and cover the cheese with a few slices of smoked salmon. Wrap the sides of the omelet onto the middle and close the lid. Switch off the heat, allow to sit 2-3 min.
5. Serve garnished with favorite greens and avocado slices.

Enjoy!

Keto Edge featured ingredient: SALMON

Among health-related properties/actions: Anti-inflammatory, supportive of cardiovascular health, antioxidant, weight regulation.

Among known active molecules/compounds: A carotenoid antioxidant, astaxanthin, gives salmon its pigment. It regulates cholesterol and is thought to work with Omega 3 fatty acids (also found in salmon) to protect brain and neurons from inflammation.

Note: Wild salmon instead of farmed is more nutritious, has better Omega 3 : Omega 6 ratios, and is less likely to have contaminants. When in doubt, it is recommended to use Omega 3 from quality Omega 3 supplements. Thus, we recommend against farm-raised salmon and prefer line/ocean caught.

Sources:
Nutrients. 2014, 6(3):1293-317.
https://www.ncbi.nlm.nih.gov/pmc/articles/PMC3967194/
J Med Food. 2014, 17(7):810-16.
https://pubmed.ncbi.nlm.nih.gov/24955642
J Atheroscler Thromb. 2000, 7(4):216-22.
https://pubmed.ncbi.nlm.nih.gov/11521685

Loaded Ground Beef Scrambled Eggs

Serves 2

Ingredients
1 tbsp lard or coconut oil
¼ cup sliced mushrooms
¼ cup diced onion
2 oz ground beef
¼ cup diced bell peppers (green, red, orange)
4 large eggs, beaten
2 tbsp crumbled feta cheese
⅛ tsp ginger powder
Salt and pepper to taste
Tomato slices and greens for garnishing

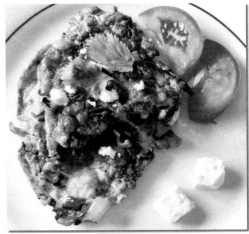

Preparation
1. In the pan, heat the oil.
2. Add the mushrooms, peppers, and onions – sauté for 5 min.
3. Add the ground beef, sauté until cooked.
4. Whisk the eggs in a bowl, add salt, pepper, ginger powder.
5. Pour the egg over the mixture in the skillet. Cook over medium heat until the egg mixture starts solidifying.
6. Sprinkle feta cheese crumbs and fold the mixture in half. Close the lid, switch off the heat, allow to sit 2-3 min.
7. Garnish with favorite greens and fresh tomatoes.

Enjoy!

Keto Edge featured ingredient: GINGER POWDER
Among health-related properties/actions: Circulatory stimulant, digestive, analgesic, anti-inflammatory, anti-pyretic (reduces fevers), antispasmodic, antimicrobial, antioxidant, relieves nausea.

Among known active molecules/compounds: [6]-Gingerol is believed to be the most abundant bioactive molecule in ginger root. Ginger is known to assist with a variety of powerful therapeutic and preventive effects used for thousands of years, to treat various symptoms from colds to cancer.

Sources:
Life Sci. 2003, 73(26):3427-37.
https://pubmed.ncbi.nlm.nih.gov/14572883
Planta Med. 2008, 74(13):1560-69.
https://pubmed.ncbi.nlm.nih.gov/18612945
J Ethnopharmacol. 2005, 96(1-2):207-10.
https://pubmed.ncbi.nlm.nih.gov/15588672
Planta Med. 2007, 73(15):1525-30.
https://pubmed.ncbi.nlm.nih.gov/18058610

Egg Salad Chicken Wraps

Serves 2

Ingredients

2 oz cooked (boiled or baked) chicken meat
4 hardboiled eggs
2 tbsp organic mayonnaise
1 tbsp lemon juice
¼ lime washed well and pureed
¼ tsp Himalayan salt
½ cup diced cilantro
4 leaves of romaine salad (or radicchio)
Lemon slices for garnish

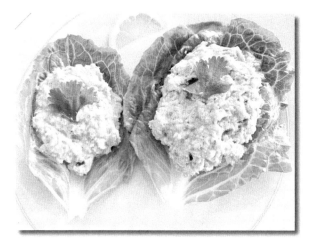

Preparation

1. In a mixer, combine hardboiled eggs, cooked chicken, mayonnaise, lemon juice, fresh lime, and salt. Puree well.
2. Transfer the content to the bowl, add the cilantro and mix well.
3. Fill each romaine leaf with the received egg salad chicken mix.
4. Serve chilled. Add lemon slices and parsley for garnish.

Enjoy!

Keto Edge featured ingredient: CILANTRO

Among health-related properties/actions: Antifungal, anti-inflammatory, antioxidant, supports cardiovascular health.

Among known active molecules/compounds: The extract of *Coriandrum Sativum* was found to have reduced skin photoaging. It was studied to lower gene expression in cancer cells, and it was shown to have antifungal properties when studied with its effects on a commonly opportunistic yeast, *Candida albicans*.

Sources:
J Med Food. 2014, 17(9):985-95.
https://www.liebertpub.com/doi/full/10.1089/jmf.2013.2999
J Cell Biochem. 2019, 120(3):3506-13.
https://www.ncbi.nlm.nih.gov/pubmed/30417420
PLoS One. 2014, 9(6):e99086.
https://journals.plos.org/plosone/article?id=10.1371/journal.pone.0099086

Italian Baked Eggs

Serves 4

Ingredients

4 tsp coconut oil
8 eggs
8 tbsp marinara sauce (lowest sugar possible!)
½ cup chopped broccoli
½ cup grated mozzarella cheese
Salt and pepper to taste
Garnish with parsley

Preparation

1. Preheat the oven to 350°F.
2. Grease 4 ramekins by placing 1 tsp coconut oil in each.
3. Break 2 eggs into each ramekin.
4. Season with salt, pepper, add 2 tbsp of marinara sauce to each.
5. Place the ramekins onto a baking sheet and bake for 10-12 min (until the yolks start hardening).
6. Divide mozzarella and top each serving.
7. Add a few pieces of broccoli, switch off the oven and let sit for another 2-3 min.
8. Serve warm.

Enjoy!

Keto Edge featured ingredient: BROCCOLI

Among health-related properties/actions: Regulates digestion, anti-inflammatory, antioxidant, cholesterol reduction, detoxification, cancer prevention.

Among known active molecules/compounds: A compound sulforaphane has been shown to reduce cancer development and recurrence and is well utilized in chemoprevention studies. Sulforaphane is an antioxidant and can activate the detoxifying enzymes in the body. It was shown to ameliorate obesity and insulin resistance in mice.

Note: When broccoli is consumed raw, it was shown to be faster absorbed and in greater bioavailability in human body.

Sources:
Drug Des Devel Ther. 2018, 12:2905-13.
https://www.ncbi.nlm.nih.gov/pmc/articles/PMC6141106/
Diabetes. 2017, 66(5):1222-36.
https://diabetes.diabetesjournals.org/content/66/5/1222
J Agric Food Chem. 2008, 56:10505-09.
https://pubs.acs.org/doi/10.1021/jf801989e

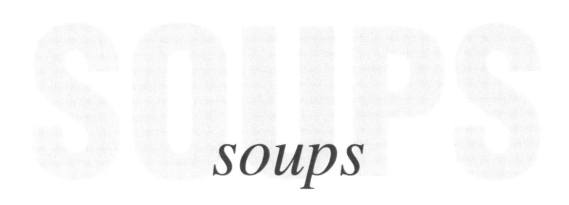

soups

Cilantro Lime Meatball Soup

Chicken or Beef Soup with Almonds

Chia Mushroom Soup

Beet Soup (Borsch)

Spinach & Tofu Soup

Cilantro Lime Meatball Soup

Serves 4

Ingredients

For Meatballs:
1 lb ground beef
½ cup finely chopped mushrooms
¼ cup parmesan cheese
¼ cup finely chopped onions
1 clove garlic, minced
½ tsp Himalayan salt
¼ tsp ground cumin
1 egg

For Soup:
1 tbsp lard (or coconut oil)
¼ cup chopped onions
1 clove garlic, minced
2 cups beef bone broth
½ cup chopped green bell pepper
1 tomato, chopped
¼ cup mushroom slices
¼ cup fresh cilantro, chopped
2 tbsp lime juice
Lime slices, for garnish

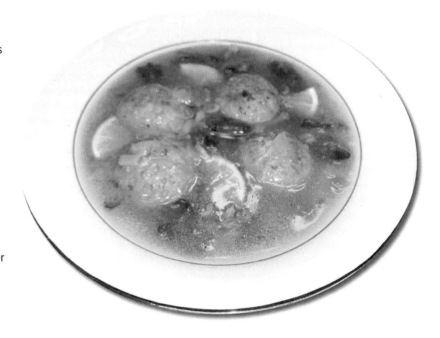

Preparation
1. Preheat the oven to 350°F.
2. In a bowl, mix ground beef, mushrooms, onions, garlic, salt, cumin, and egg. Shape the mixture into meatballs, place on the baking sheet, and bake for 20 min or until cooked.
3. In a large saucepan, heat the lard.
4. Add the onions, bell peppers, tomatoes, garlic, salt, and sauté for 3 min.
5. Add the broth and bring to a boil. Reduce the heat and simmer until the meatballs are ready.
6. Add the meatballs, bring to a brief boil, and add the lime juice. Switch off the heat.
7. Add cilantro and lime slices, allow to sit for 5 min with a closed lid.
8. Ladle into bowls with several lime slices in each portion.

Enjoy!

Keto Edge featured ingredient: CUMIN

Among health-related properties/actions: Antioxidant, anticancer, digestive regulation, blood sugar control, antibacterial, anti-inflammatory, regulates weight loss, boosts memory.

Among known active molecules/compounds: Beta-pinene, found in many essential oils and well represented in cumin, shows gastroprotective, anticonvulsant, antioxidative, and neuroprotective effects.

Note: Cumin can suppress testosterone levels if consumed in excess.

Sources:
J Pharmacy. 2016, 6(6):45-46.
http://iosrphr.org/papers/v6i6V2/G066024665.pdf
Biomolecules. 2019, 9(11):738.
https://www.ncbi.nlm.nih.gov/pmc/articles/PMC6920849/
JMPS. 2018, 6(2):232-36.
http://www.plantsjournal.com/archives/2018/vol6issue2/PartD/6-2-28-858.pdf

Chicken or Beef Soup with Almonds

Serves 2-4

Ingredients

1 large boneless chicken breast (or can use beef)
4 tbsp olive oil
1 celery stalk
3 cups chicken broth
½ cup ground almonds
2 tbsp lemon juice
Salt and pepper
3 stems green onions, chopped

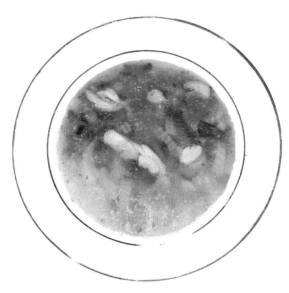

Preparation

1.   Cut each chicken breast into strips, slice thinly to give shreds of meat.
2.   Heat the oil in a frying pan, add the chicken and toss until almost cooked.
3.   Add the celery, stir well.
4.   In a boiling pan, heat the chicken broth, add the lemon juice, salt and pepper.
5.   Transfer the contents from the frying pan into the boiling pan. Bring the mixture to a boil and let simmer, uncovered, stirring occasionally.
6.   Add the ground almonds and chopped green onions, continue to cook for additional 1-2 min. Serve warm.

Enjoy!

Keto Edge featured ingredient: ALMOND
Among health-related properties/actions: Antioxidant, cholesterol lowering action, regulation of the digestive tract, immunostimulant, aphrodisiac.

Among known active molecules/compounds: Almond skin flavonoids (ASL) were shown to protect cholesterol in the body from oxidation. This effect is observed even longer when ASLs are combined with vitamin C (which comes from lemon juice in this recipe).

Note: Did you know that almond is technically not a nut? It is an edible drupe, with a tough fibrous rind that surrounds the stone or "shell" and the seed or "nut."

Sources:
Article "Legumes, Nuts & Seeds."
https://faculty.ucr.edu/~legneref/botany/legunuts.htm
J Nutr. 2005, 135(6):1366-73.
https://academic.oup.com/jn/article/135/6/1366/4663832
J Nutr Biochem. 2007, 18(12):785-94.
https://www.ncbi.nlm.nih.gov/pubmed/17475462

Chia Mushroom Soup

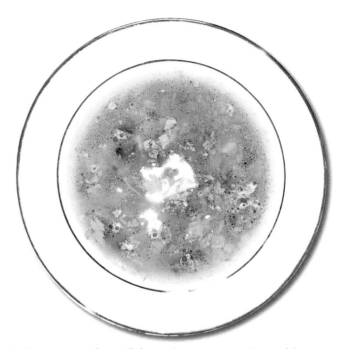

Serves 2-4

Ingredients

8 oz mushrooms, chopped
1 medium onion, chopped
1 stalk of celery, chopped
3 garlic cloves, crushed
2 tbsp butter or olive oil
1 quart vegetable stock (or water)
½ tsp thyme powder
½ cup chia seeds
Salt and pepper to taste
4 tbsp sour cream
Garnish with parsley, chopped

Preparation

1. In a large pan, melt the butter.
2. Add the mushrooms, onion, celery and cook stirring constantly until the onion starts turning golden.
3. Add the garlic and stir another 1 min.
4. In a boiling pan, add the vegetable stock, add thyme and a pinch of salt, and bring to a boil. Add chia seeds.
5. Transfer the content from the large pan into the boiling pan. Bring to a boil, then reduce the heat to medium and allow to simmer for 15 min.
6. Remove the pan, allow to cool briefly. Serve topped with a spoon of sour cream, garnish with parsley.

Enjoy!

Keto Edge featured ingredient: PARSLEY

Among health-related properties/actions: Rich in nutrients (such as vitamin A, C, K), antioxidant, antiviral, antibacterial, blood pressure reduction, anti-inflammatory. Supports heart health, supports kidney health, supports healthy blood sugar, supports bone health, can aid with digestive system health, anticancer.

Among known active molecules/compounds: A flavonoid molecule found in parsley, apigenin, has been repeatedly shown to have strong anticancer properties. As an example, apigenin was found to effectively treat breast cancer. When apigenin was combined with green tea, the rate of colon cancer was successfully reduced in patients.

Sources:
Cell Biosci. 2017, 7:50.
https://www.ncbi.nlm.nih.gov/pmc/articles/PMC5629766/
"Breast Cancer Effectively Treated," Article, New Bureau University of Missouri.
https://munewsarchives.missouri.edu/news-releases/2012/0515-breast-cancer-effectively-treated-with-chemical-found-in-celery-parsley-and-spice-by-mu-researchers/
Int J Mol Sci. 2019, 20(6):1305.
https://www.ncbi.nlm.nih.gov/pmc/articles/PMC6472148/

Beet Soup (Borsch)

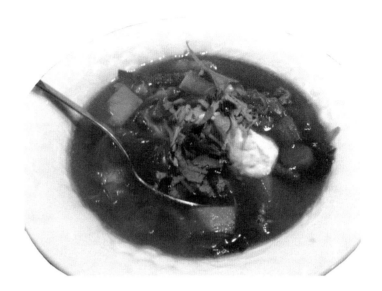

Serves 2-4

Ingredients
½ pound ground beef
1 onion, chopped
2 parsnips, peeled and cut into thin slices
1 small celery root, chopped
1 turnip, chopped
1 medium beet, chopped
1 medium carrot, chopped
1 medium tomato, chopped
1 cup chopped cabbage
4 tbsp olive oil
3 ½ cups low-sodium beef broth or
    homemade stock
3 cups water
¼ tsp fresh-ground black pepper
1 ½ tsp Himalayan salt
¼ cup sour cream
Garnish with parsley, cilantro, or dill

Preparation
1. In a large saucepan, heat the oil over moderately low heat.
2. Add the onion and cook, stirring occasionally, until translucent, about 5 minutes.
3. Add the parsnips, celery root, turnip, and 1 teaspoon of salt. Cover and cook until the vegetables start to soften, about 5 minutes.
4. Add the ground beef and cook another 5 min.
5. Add the beets, carrots, tomatoes, cabbage, broth, water, the remaining ½ teaspoon salt, and the pepper. Bring to a boil. Reduce the heat and simmer, uncovered, until the vegetables are tender, about 15 minutes.
6. Serve topped with the garnish of choice and sour cream.

Enjoy!

Keto Edge featured ingredient: BEETS
Among health-related properties/actions: Lowering blood pressure, anti-inflammatory, regulates digestive tract, immune booster, aphrodisiac, aids with eyesight.

Among known active molecules/compounds: Beets (sometimes referred to as beetroot) are a rich source of betanin, a multi-functional phytochemical molecule shown to inhibit lipid oxidation. Betanin pigments have been studied in lab to lessen tumor cell growth through various mechanisms, including the inhibition of pro-inflammatory enzymes, inhibition of lipid oxidation. Betanin effects have been researched for chemoprevention.

Sources:
Molecules. 2019, 24(3):458. https://www.ncbi.nlm.nih.govpubmed/30696032
Mol Nutr Food Res. 2015, 59(1):36-47. https://www.ncbi.nlm.nih.gov/pubmed/25178819
Anticancer Agents Med Chem. 2011, 11(3):280-84. https://www.ncbi.nlm.nih.gov/pubmed/21434853
Free Radic Res. 2007, 41(3):335-41. https://www.ncbi.nlm.nih.gov/pubmed/17364963

Spinach & Tofu Soup

Serves 2-4

Ingredients

8 oz tofu, sliced in cubes
4 ½ oz fresh spinach leaves, cut or shredded
3 cups vegetable broth
1 tsp light soy sauce
2 tbsp sesame oil
2 tbsp MCT oil
¼ tsp Himalayan salt
¼ tsp black pepper

Preparation
1. In a pan, heat the vegetable broth to a boil.
2. Add the tofu and soy sauce, return to a boil and simmer for 3-4 minutes.
3. Add the sesame oil, MCT oil, and spinach, simmer another 1-2 min while stirring.
4. Add salt and pepper to taste. Serve hot.

Enjoy!

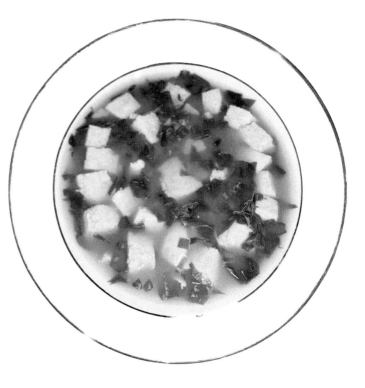

Keto Edge featured ingredient: SESAME OIL
Among health-related properties/actions: Antiviral, antibacterial, antioxidant, antiaging, anti-inflammatory, anticancer, anti-diabetes.

Among known active molecules/compounds: Sesamin has been studied in the context of regulating blood pressure, prevention of hyperlipidemia, hypertension, and carcinogenesis through an unknown mechanism. Sesamin was shown to have anti-inflammatory effects and reduce photo-damage in lab studies in skin cells.

Sources:
Molecules. 2019, 24(24):4426.
https://www.ncbi.nlm.nih.gov/pmc/articles/PMC6943436/
Biomolecules. 2019, 12:9(9).
https://www.ncbi.nlm.nih.gov/pubmed/31547364
Article "Sesame seeds," Netmed.
https://www.netmeds.com/health-library/post/sesame-seeds-tiny-huge-benefits

meat & fish

Beefy Cauliflower & Almond Stir-Fry

Curry Beef Meatballs

Liver Pancakes

Kielbasa and Sauerkraut

Chicken Sausage with Zucchini Stir-Fry

Ginger Coconut Chicken

Lemon Pepper Chicken Legs (or Tenders)

Beefy Broccoli & Walnut Stir-Fry

Steak with Creamy Vegetable Topping

Spiced Beef Tips

Salmon Patties with Avocado

Salmon with Cucumber Sauce

Beefy Cauliflower & Almond Stir-Fry

Serves 2-4

Ingredients

2 tbsp lard (can substitute with ghee or olive oil)
3 cloves garlic, minced
1 small onion, minced
1 lb ground beef
16 oz cauliflower
½ cup almonds
¼ tsp turmeric powder
¼ tsp black pepper

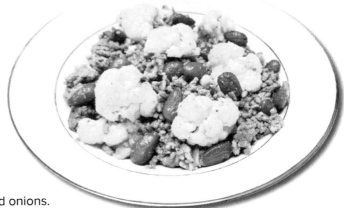

Preparation

1. In a large skillet, heat the lard and add garlic and onions.
2. Add beef. Cook until beef is well browned, stirring occasionally.
3. Stir in almonds, add turmeric powder and black pepper, cook for additional 5 min.
4. Add cauliflower, cook for 5 min more.

Enjoy!

Keto Edge featured ingredient: TURMERIC POWDER

Among health-related properties/actions: Antioxidant, antibiotic, anti-inflammatory, digestive, anti-obesity, anticarcinogenic.

Among known active molecules/compounds: The main known active ingredient in turmeric, curcumin, has been studied vastly for its antioxidant, anticancer effects; it is well known for its anti-inflammatory properties that are comparable to known anti-inflammatory agents.

Note: Curcumin bioavailability is increased when it is combined with black pepper.

Sources:
Herbal Medicine: Biomolecular and Clinical Aspects. 2011, Ch. 13.
https://www.ncbi.nlm.nih.gov/books/NBK92752/
Mol Med Rep. 2012, 6(6):1267-70.
https://www.ncbi.nlm.nih.gov/pubmed/23023821
Foods. 2017, 6(10): 92.
https://www.ncbi.nlm.nih.gov/pmc/articles/PMC5664031/
Planta Med. 1998, 64(4):353-6.
https://pubmed.ncbi.nlm.nih.gov/9619120

Curry Beef Meatballs

Serves 2-4

Ingredients

For meatballs:
1 lb ground beef
½ cup finely chopped mushrooms
¼ cup parmesan cheese
¼ cup finely chopped onions
1 clove garlic, minced
½ tsp Himalayan salt
¼ tsp ground cumin
1 egg

For sauce:
¼ cup lard or coconut oil
½ cup onions, chopped
4 cloves of garlic, minced
1 tbsp peeled and grated fresh ginger (or marinated)
½ cup green bell peppers, chopped
2 tbsp garam masala mix
4 tbsp tomato sauce
1 tbsp turmeric powder
1 medium tomato, chopped
1 tsp Himalayan salt
2 tbsp lemon juice
Garnish with fresh cilantro

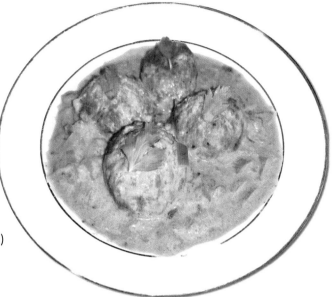

Preparation
1. Preheat the oven to 350°F.
2. In a bowl, mix ground beef, mushrooms, onions, garlic, salt, cumin, and egg. Shape the mixture into meatballs, place on the baking sheet, and bake for 20 min or until cooked.
3. In a large skillet, heat the lard. Add the onions, garlic, ginger, bell peppers, and sauté for 3-5 min.
4. Add the garam masala mix, tomato sauce, turmeric, and stir well.
5. Mix in the chopped tomatoes and salt. Simmer on medium heat for 10 min.
6. Add lemon juice and bring in the cooked meatballs, mixing them with the sauce and allowing to simmer for another 5-10 min.
7. Serve with chopped cilantro.

Enjoy the strong flavor of mixed spices in this meal!

Keto Edge featured ingredient: CLOVES (in Garam Masala)
Garam Masala content has many variations and is generally comprised of well over a dozen of various spices, including cloves.

Among health-related properties/actions: Antiseptic, antibacterial, antifungal, and antiviral properties, researched for potential anticancer effects.

Among known active molecules/compounds: Ethyl acetate extract of cloves (EAEC), with Oleanolic acid being one of the bioactive components, shows anti-inflammatory effects and is used for regulating healthy liver metabolism and for regulating blood sugar.

Sources:
Oncol Res. 2014, 21(5): 247-59.
https://www.ncbi.nlm.nih.gov/pmc/articles/PMC4132639/
Molecules. 2013, 18(3):3060-71.
https://www.ncbi.nlm.nih.gov/pubmed/23470335
J Ethnopharmacol. 1995, 49(2):57-68.
https://www.ncbi.nlm.nih.gov/pubmed/8847885

Liver Pancakes

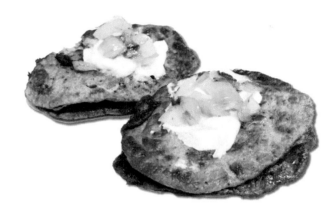

Serves 2-3

Ingredients
12 oz beef or chicken liver, pureed
1 egg
2 tbsp almond flour
2 tbsp lard or coconut oil
1 medium onion, chopped
¼ tsp salt
¼ tsp black pepper
4 tbsp mayonnaise
1 garlic clove, crushed

Preparation
1. In a mixing bowl, mix the pureed liver with the egg, almond flour, salt, and black pepper.
2. In a frying pan, heat the lard, turn the heat to medium, and carefully ladle out the liver mixture into pancake portions to cook on both sides.
3. Once finished, collect the pancakes and add the onion (chopped) onto the frying pan, sauté until golden. Let the pancakes cool off.
4. In a mixing bowl, mix the crushed garlic clove with the mayonnaise.
5. Place a pancake onto a serving plate, cover with the mayonnaise mixture, and add another pancake. Garnish with the mayonnaise mixture topped with the golden onions.

Serve warm or chilled and enjoy!

Keto Edge featured ingredient: LIVER

Among health-related properties/actions: Liver is a remarkable organ that is highly nutrient-dense and with large amounts of B vitamins, as well as high doses of vitamin A, copper, iron — all important in hundreds of metabolic processes in the body. Liver provides quality protein and has fewer calories than most meats.

Among known active molecules/compounds: Choline is a vitamin-like nutrient (considered essential) and a methyl donor involved in many physiological processes including epigenetic regulation, transport of lipids, and normal metabolism. Choline is important for brain development, memory, nervous system functions at large, and liver function.

Note: Liver is not advised to be consumed heavily during pregnancy (due to high vitamin A) and in cases with gout type of arthritis.

Sources:
Article "Choline." Oregon State University website.
https://lpi.oregonstate.edu/mic/other-nutrients/choline
Nutr Rev. 2009, 67(11):615-23.
https://www.ncbi.nlm.nih.gov/pmc/articles/PMC2782876/
Article "Vitamin A." NIH Office of Dietary Supplements.
https://ods.od.nih.gov/factsheets/VitaminA-HealthProfessional/
Article "Choline." NIH Office of Dietary Supplements.
https://ods.od.nih.gov/factsheets/Choline-HealthProfessional/

Kielbasa and Sauerkraut

Serves 2-3

Ingredients

16 oz sauerkraut
1 lb polish kielbasa (beef, pork, or turkey)
4 tbsp olive oil
1-2 green onion stalks, chopped

Preparation

1. In a medium saucepan, bring the sauerkraut to a boil.
2. Slice the sausage into rings and add onto the pan. Add the olive oil and simmer over low heat until heated through (5-10 min).
3. Add the green onion stalks to the contents of the pan. Close the lid, switch off the heat and let stand for 1-2 min. Serve warm.

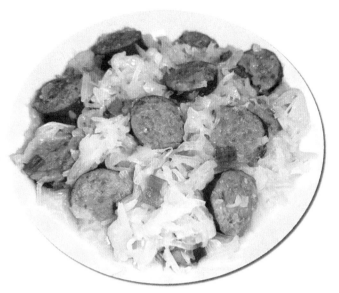

Enjoy!

Keto Edge featured ingredient: SAUERKRAUT

Among health-related properties/actions: Improves digestion, can help with regulating weight, boosts immune system, supports bone health, may help with regulating blood pressure, researched for anticancer effects.

Among known active molecules/compounds: Kaempferol is one of the flavonoids found to remain stable in the cabbage fiber over the fermentation process. It participates in the properties described above and has been linked to decreasing the risk of several cancers, including skin, liver, and colon.

Note: When buying commercial sauerkraut, it is best to obtain non-pasteurized, no-sugars added product without preservatives.

Sources:
JAMA. 2012, 307(18):1959-69.
https://jamanetwork.com/journals/jama/fullarticle/1151505
J Agric Food Chem. 2002, 50(23):6798-803.
https://pubs.acs.org/doi/10.1021/jf0109017
Molecules. 2019, 24(12):2277.
https://www.ncbi.nlm.nih.gov/pmc/articles/PMC6631472/
Biotechnol Res Int. 2014, 2014:250424.
https://www.ncbi.nlm.nih.gov/pmc/articles/PMC4058509/

Chicken Sausage with Zucchini Stir-Fry

Serves 2

Ingredients

1 lb chicken sausages (flavored or plain)
1 lb zucchini, sliced or chopped
1 medium onion, chopped in cubes
1 tsp minced garlic
¼ cup water
4 tbsp olive oil
¼ tsp ginger powder
¼ tsp thyme powder
¼ tsp Himalayan salt
Fresh greens if desired

Preparation

1. Heat a large pan over medium heat, add water and oil. Stir in minced garlic and ginger powder and cook until fragrant.
2. Add the sausages and allow to absorb the flavor from the pan by turning to 4 sides until cooked (optional – chicken sausages can be grilled instead).
3. Add chopped onion cubes, cook until slightly softened (2 min).
4. Add zucchini, mix with the content on the pan. Add thyme powder and let simmer until fragrant.
5. Garnish with fresh greens and serve warm.

Enjoy!

Keto Edge featured ingredient: THYME

Among health-related properties/actions: Digestive, antibacterial, decongestant, circulatory stimulant, boosts immune system, antioxidant.

Among known active molecules/compounds: Rosmarinic acid and flavonoid derivatives found in thyme classify it as high in the antioxidant activity. Rosmarinic acid effects observed in relation to human body are numerous, including the anticancer effects, immunity boosting, antioxidant effects, and antimicrobial activities.

Sources:
Appl Microbiol Biotechnol. 2018, 102(18):7775-93.
https://link.springer.com/article/10.1007%2Fs00253-018-9223-y
Int J Mol Sci. 2019, 20(7):1749.
https://www.ncbi.nlm.nih.gov/pmc/articles/PMC6479806/
Herbal Medicine: Biomolecular and Clinical Aspects. 2011. Ch.17
https://www.ncbi.nlm.nih.gov/books/NBK92774/

Ginger Coconut Chicken

Serves 4

Ingredients

4-6 bone-in, skin-on chicken thighs
3 tbsp peeled and grated fresh ginger
2 tbsp minced garlic
1 (¾ and ¼) tsp Himalayan salt
2 tbsp lime juice
½ cup broth of choice or water
1 tomato, medium, chopped
3 cups cilantro
3 tbsp coconut oil
½ cup cashew halves
1 cup coconut milk
2-4 oz of medium-hard cheese

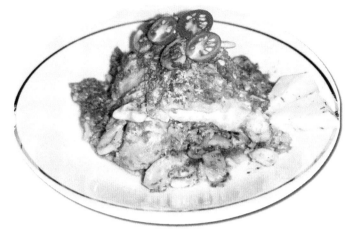

Preparation

1. In a mixer, chop together the ginger, garlic, lime juice, ¼ tbsp salt, 2 tbsp broth (or water). Apply the combined mixture onto chicken thighs in a separate bowl (can be marinated in the fridge overnight if desired).
2. In a mixer/blender, add tomato, cilantro, ¾ tsp of salt, 2 tbsp of broth. Puree these ingredients.
3. In a skillet, heat the oil and place the marinated chicken, turning occasionally, until lightly golden (~10 min).
4. Add the remaining broth. Pour the tomato-cilantro mix onto the chicken. Cook, stirring often, until the sauce starts thickening.
5. Add the coconut milk and cashews and bring to a boil. Then lower the heat to medium and cook until the chicken is no longer pink inside (~10 min).
6. Serve with the tomato-cilantro reduction and cheese of preference on the side (we used Parmesan dill cheese).

Enjoy!

Keto Edge featured ingredient: LIME JUICE
Among health-related properties/actions: Antimicrobial, immune booster, antioxidant.

Among known active molecules/compounds: Lime contains a natural flavonoid hesperidin, which was shown for its antioxidant abilities. It was also found to assist with combatting cancers including breast, lung, liver, and colon cancer.

Note: Based on numerous studies of various active compounds such as hesperidin, not every promising compound makes it to the treatment studies due to stability. Consuming healthy foods and leading a healthy lifestyle is another way to assist the body with reducing aches and disease risks.

Sources:
Pharmacogn Rev. 2016, 10(20):118-22.
https://www.ncbi.nlm.nih.gov/pmc/articles/PMC5214556/
Front Pharmacol. 2017, 8:420.
https://www.ncbi.nlm.nih.gov/pmc/articles/PMC5491624/
Nutrients. 2016, 8(11):698.
https://www.ncbi.nlm.nih.gov/pmc/articles/PMC5133085/#B222-nutrients-08-00698

Lemon Pepper Chicken Legs (or Tenders)

Serves 2-4

Ingredients

¼ cup coconut oil
1 tbsp minced garlic
2 lemons, sliced
4 chicken legs or boneless skinless chicken
   tenders
2 tbsp lemon pepper seasoning
2 tsp Himalayan salt
1 tsp black peppercorns, for garnish
Chopped greens (parsley or oregano) for garnish

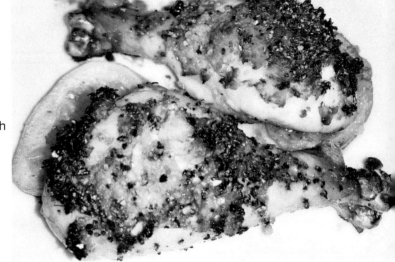

Preparation

1. Preheat the oven to 400°F.
2. Make the lemon sauce: Place the oil and garlic in a small bowl. Grate the zest of one of the lemons and add 2 tsp of the zest to the bowl. Juice the zested lemon and add the juice to the bowl. Stir well.
3. Cut the 2nd lemon into thin slices and arrange on a baking sheet. Season all sides of the chicken strips with the lemon pepper seasoning and salt. Place the chicken on top of the lemon slices. Bake for 20 min.
4. Serve garnished with peppercorns and fresh parsley to taste.

Enjoy!

Keto Edge featured ingredient: BLACK PEPPER/PEPPERCORN

Among health-related properties/actions: Supports digestion, regulates blood pressure and cholesterol levels. The antioxidant, anticancer and anti-inflammatory activities are being shown and researched.

Among known active molecules/compounds: Piperine, the most important compound of black pepper, is attributed with the effects observed from black pepper.

Note: If using crushed or ground black pepper, it begins to lose flavor after about 4 months.

Sources:
Nat Prod Commun. 2010, 5(8):1253-57.
https://pubmed.ncbi.nlm.nih.gov/20839630
Article "Peppercorn and Pepper Storage and Selection." The Spruce Eats website.
https://www.thespruceeats.com/peppercorn-and-pepper-storage-and-selection-1807792
Adv Exp Med Biol. 2016, 928:173-84.
https://pubmed.ncbi.nlm.nih.gov/27671817

Beefy Broccoli & Walnut Stir-Fry

Serves 2-3

Ingredients

2 tbsp lard (can substitute with ghee or olive oil)
3 cloves garlic, minced
1 small onion, minced
1 lb ground beef
16 oz broccoli
½ cup walnut pieces or halves
¼ tsp ginger powder

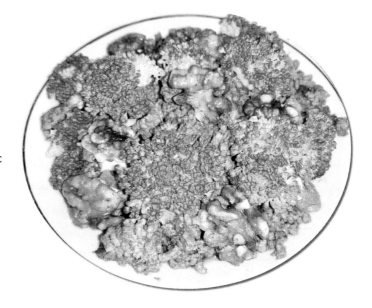

Preparation

1. In a large skillet, heat the lard and add garlic and onions.
2. Add beef. Cook until beef is well browned, stirring occasionally.
3. Stir in walnuts, add ginger powder, cook for additional 5 min.
4. Add broccoli, cook for additional 5 min.

Enjoy!

Keto Edge featured ingredient: WALNUTS

Among health-related properties/actions: Rich in antioxidants, a good source of Omega 3, boosting immunity, reducing inflammation, regulates weight, may reduce risk of some cancers.

Among known active molecules/compounds: Walnuts contain some of the most important polyphenols, with ellagitannins being studied to aid in cancer, cardiovascular, and neurodegenerative diseases.

Sources:
Crit Rev Food Sci Nutr. 2017, 57(16):3373-83.
https://pubmed.ncbi.nlm.nih.gov/26713565
Toxins (Basel). 2018, 10(11):469.
https://www.ncbi.nlm.nih.gov/pmc/articles/PMC6266065/
Crit Rev Food Sci Nutr. 2016, 56(8):1231-41.
https://pubmed.ncbi.nlm.nih.gov/25747270

Steak with Creamy Vegetable Topping

Serves 3-4

Ingredients
2 ribeye steaks - 1 lb each
½ cup red wine
½ cup heavy cream

Vegetable topping:
¼ cup coconut oil to sauté
½ cup onions
½ cup peppers (green red yellow)
½ cup mushrooms
Garnish with oregano leaves

Spices:
1 tbsp ground black pepper
1 tbsp ground red pepper
1 tbsp coarse salt
1 tbsp ground paprika
2 cloves garlic minced
Mix all in a small container

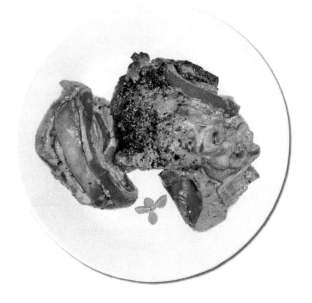

Preparation
Use ⅔ of the spices mixture for vegetables while sautéing. Use ⅓ of this mixture for meat while broiling.

1. Preheat the oven to broil at 525°F.
2. Place steaks in a broiler. Broil for approximately 5-6 min per side (following the first 6 min, remove the steaks from the oven, flip to the other side, apply half of ⅓ of the spices mixture).
3. To sauté vegetable mix: In a frying pan, heat the oil, add the vegetables, onions, and mushrooms, mix on high heat, then reduce to medium heat.
4. Add ⅔ of the spices mixture, red wine, heavy cream. Stir well and sauté on high heat until the mixture is bubbling (5-7 min).
5. Reduce to lower heat to continue reduction until the mixture is thickened and creamy.
6. Remove from heat. Sprinkle the steak with the remaining (half of ⅓) mixture of spices. Garnish with oregano leaves.

Enjoy!

Keto Edge featured ingredient: PAPRIKA
Among health-related properties/actions: Thought to improve vision, improve cholesterol levels, reduce inflammation, have antioxidant and anticancer effects.

Among known active molecules/compounds: Capsanthin and capsaicin found in paprika are studied for the above mentioned actions.

Sources:
Cancer Lett. 2001, 172(2):103-09.
https://pubmed.ncbi.nlm.nih.gov/11566483
Anticancer Res. 2016, 36(3):837-43.
https://pubmed.ncbi.nlm.nih.gov/26976969
Molecules. 2016, 21(8):966.
https://www.ncbi.nlm.nih.gov/pmc/articles/PMC6272969/

Spiced Beef Tips

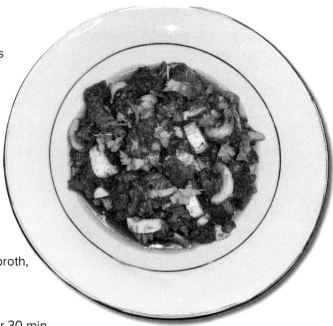

Serves 4

Ingredients

1 boneless sirloin or boneless ribeye (~ 1 lb), cut in cubes
2 stalks of celery, chopped
¼ cup onions, chopped
4 cloves garlic, minced
2 cups marinara sauce
1 cup beef bone broth
½ tsp Moroccan spice
½ tsp ground black pepper
½ tsp sea salt
Garnish with fresh oregano or thyme

Preparation

1. In a slow cooker (4-quart), mix the marinara sauce, broth, onions, Moroccan spice, black pepper, salt.
2. Add the meat cubes. Cover and let cook on low for 4 hours or until the meat is tender.
3. Add the chopped celery and garlic, cook for another 30 min.
4. Serve with the sauce from the slow cooker.
5. Garnish with fresh oregano or thyme if desired.

Enjoy!

Keto Edge featured ingredient: ALLSPICE (in Moroccan spice)
Among health-related properties/actions: Allspice can relieve pain, ease stomach upset, benefit skin and hair, and kill bacteria and fungus. It is researched for treating cancer and hypertension.

Among known active molecules/compounds: Eugenol and quercetin in Allspice are studied for reducing inflammation, regulating cardiovascular health, and showing antitumor effects.

Sources:
Article "Allspice. Antioxidant Properties of Spices, Herbs and Other Sources by Denys Charles. pp. 145-150.
https://link.springer.com/chapter/10.1007/978-1-4614-4310-0_6
Curr Drug Targets. 2012, 13(14):1900-06.
https://pubmed.ncbi.nlm.nih.gov/23140298
Oncol Rep. 2017, 38(2):819-28.
https://www.ncbi.nlm.nih.gov/pmc/articles/PMC5561933/

Salmon Patties with Avocado

Serves 2-3

Ingredients

1 lb Atlantic salmon, chopped
2 eggs
1 medium onion, chopped
¼ tsp Himalayan salt
¼ tsp Thyme spice
6 romaine lettuce leaves
1 avocado, pitted and sliced
2 tbsp mayonnaise
1 tbsp chopped parsley (or dill)
2 tsp lemon juice
2 tbsp coconut oil
½ cup water

Preparation

1. In a bowl, mix chopped salmon and onions with the eggs. Add salt, and thyme spice. Mix well and form into six round patties.
2. In a large cast-iron skillet, heat the oil with water. Add the patties and cook for 3 min or until they turn lightly golden. Flip and cook until golden brown on both sides.
3. For the sauce, mix the mayonnaise with lemon juice and chopped parsley. Add a pinch of salt if desired.
4. Serve the patties on lettuce leaves, top with a spoon of the sauce, garnished with a slice of lemon if desired. Add the sliced avocado.

Enjoy!

Keto Edge featured ingredient: AVOCADO
Among health-related properties/actions: Nutritious superfood, regulation of cholesterol and triglyceride levels, loaded with powerful antioxidants, researched for cancer prevention.

Among known active molecules/compounds: With many cancer preventing nutrients, vitamins, and phytochemicals, avocado was researched for chemoprevention purposes.

Sources:
J Exp Ther Oncol. 2011, 9(3):221-30.
https://pubmed.ncbi.nlm.nih.gov/22070054
J Nutr Biochem. 2005, 16(1):23-30.
https://pubmed.ncbi.nlm.nih.gov/15629237
Crit Rev Food Sci Nutr. 2013, 53(7):738-50.
https://pubmed.ncbi.nlm.nih.gov/2363893

Salmon with Cucumber Sauce

Serves 2-3

Ingredients

½ cup water
2 tbsp olive oil
½ teaspoon allspice
¼ teaspoon black pepper
¼ teaspoon ground rosemary
1 lb Atlantic salmon fillets
½ cup chopped cucumber
⅓ cup yogurt
2 tbsp sliced green or regular onion
2 tbsp mayonnaise
2 tbsp chopped cilantro
1 tsp mustard
2 cups shredded lettuce

Preparation

1. In a large skillet, combine water, olive oil, allspice, black pepper and rosemary. Mix and bring to hot.
2. Place the salmon fillets onto the skillet with the mixture, bring the heat to medium-low. Cover and simmer 8-10 min or until salmon starts flaking.
3. Remove the salmon and refrigerate, if desired, to serve cold.
4. In a bowl, combine cucumber, yogurt, onion, mayonnaise, cilantro, and mustard.
5. Place salmon fillets on lettuce-covered plates, pour the sauce over salmon and serve.

Enjoy!

Keto Edge featured ingredient: GROUND ROSEMARY

Among health-related properties/actions: Traditionally used to improve digestion, alleviate muscle pain, boost the immune and circulatory system, improve memory, promote hair growth.

Among known active molecules/compounds: Crude ethanolic rosemary extract (RO) was shown to inhibit the growth of human leukemia and breast carcinoma cells in lab.

Note: Adding rosemary to high-heat frying may reduce the formation of cancer-causing agents (heterocyclic amines).

Sources:
Oncol Rep. 2017, 17(6):1525-31.
https://pubmed.ncbi.nlm.nih.gov/17487414
Biosci Biotechnol Biochem. 2007, 71(9):2223-32.
https://pubmed.ncbi.nlm.nih.gov/17827696
J Food Sci. 2006, 71(8):C469-73.
https://onlinelibrary.wiley.com/doi/abs/10.1111/j.1750-3841.2006.00149.x

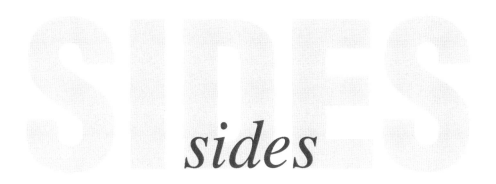

sides

Eggplant Pancakes

Salt-Roasted Turnip with Tomato and Goat Cheese

Fried Cauliflower

Stir-Fried Mushroom & Broccoli with Coconut and Walnuts

Roasted Purple Cabbage

Sautéed Parsnip Mushrooms

Brussels Sprouts and Bacon

Radicchio Eggplant Ragout

Eggplant Pancakes

Serves 2-4

Ingredients
4 tbsp olive oil
1 large eggplant
2-4 tbsp almond flour
1 egg
2 tbsp heavy cream
Salt and pepper to taste
2 garlic cloves
2 medium tomatoes (or 12 oz of grape tomatoes)
2 tbsp organic mayonnaise

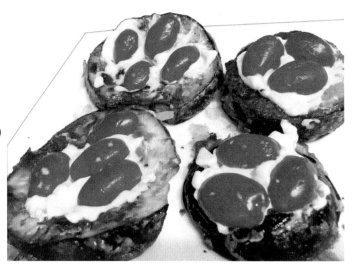

Preparation
1. Whisk an egg with heavy cream, salt and pepper.
2. Slice the eggplant into circles.
3. In a frying pan, heat the oil.
4. Dip the eggplant slices into almond flour and then into whisked egg, followed by laying onto the frying pan. Cook until golden on both sides.
5. Remove the eggplant pancakes from the pan and drain on paper towels.
6. Crush the garlic cloves and mix with mayonnaise. Add the mixture onto the prepared eggplant pancakes, top with slices of tomato (or halves of grape tomatoes).

Enjoy!

Keto Edge featured ingredient: GARLIC

Among health-related properties/actions: Antimicrobial, anthelminthic, immune booster, regulates cholesterol and blood pressure, regulates digestion, circulatory stimulant, anticancer.

Among known active molecules/compounds: Garlic contains sulfur compounds such allicin, which is known to lower blood pressure, regulate cholesterol thereby assisting with heart health. It is also known to have cancer-fighting effects with various cancer research studies including colon and stomach.

Note: It is best to use fresh garlic. If using garlic made in oil at home, use it promptly (with storage, it can host the growth of botulinum bacteria that produce toxins without changing taste or smell of oil, these bacteria can affect the nervous system and cause botulism).

Sources:
J Sci Food Agricult. 2012, 92:9.
https://onlinelibrary.wiley.com/doi/abs/10.1002/jsfa.5557
Maturitas. 2010, 67(2):144-50.
https://www.maturitas.org/article/S0378-5122(10)00227-6/fulltext
Eur J Clin Nutr. 2013, 67(1):64-70.
https://www.ncbi.nlm.nih.gov/pmc/articles/PMC3561616/
Article "Stinking facts about garlic." Michigan State University, 2015.
https://www.canr.msu.edu/news/stinking_facts_about_garlic
Biomolecules. 2020, 10(1):105. https://www.mdpi.com/2218-273X/10/1/105/htm

Salt-Roasted Turnip with Tomato and Goat Cheese

Serves 2-4

Ingredients

4 medium turnips
1 medium onion
12 oz grape tomatoes (or 2 medium tomatoes)
2 oz goat cheese, softened
¼ cup extra-virgin olive oil
Freshly ground black pepper, ginger powder,
       kosher (coarse) salt or Himalayan salt
2 sprigs of fresh oregano leaves

Preparation

1. Cut the turnips, onions, and tomatoes into rings.
2. In a large skillet, heat the oil and add turnip rings topped with the onion rings, allow to soften (place the lid on the skillet).
3. Sprinkle the tops with black pepper and ginger.
4. Top with tomato rings. Allow to simmer on low heat until turnip ring edges start turning golden.
5. Top with a piece of goat cheese (or cream cheese). Allow to simmer another 5 min.
6. On the plate, garnish each piece with fresh oregano leaves. Serve warm or chilled.

Enjoy!

Keto Edge featured ingredient: TURNIP

Among health-related properties/actions: Aiding with digestive tract, regulating weight, lowering blood pressure, antioxidant, antimicrobial, anticancer.

Among known active molecules/compounds: Phytochemicals such as indole-3-carbinol, sulforaphane, and di-indolmethane are among those studied for various health benefits including anticancer properties.

Sources:
J Food Sci. 2019, 84(1):19-30.
https://pubmed.ncbi.nlm.nih.gov/30561035-
Br J Pharmacol. 2011, 164(1):145-58.
https://www.ncbi.nlm.nih.gov/pmc/articles/PMC3171867/
Nutr Rev. 2016, 74(7):432-43.
https://www.ncbi.nlm.nih.gov/pmc/articles/PMC5059820/

Fried Cauliflower

Serves 2-4

Ingredients

12 oz cauliflower, chop into bite sized pieces
(~ ½ of a large head of cauliflower)
Olive oil for frying (as needed)

Egg Wash:
2 large eggs, whisked
4 tbsp heavy cream

Breading:
1 cup superfine blanched almond flour
1 tsp garlic powder
¼ tsp Himalayan salt
¼ tsp black pepper
¼ tsp turmeric
2-3 stems of parsley

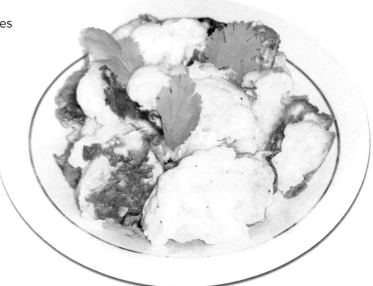

Preparation
1. In a medium bowl, whisk together almond flour, garlic powder, black pepper, salt, and turmeric. Set aside.
2. In a small bowl, whisk eggs with heavy cream. Set aside.
3. In a frying pan, heat the oil.
4. Dip a piece of cauliflower into the almond flour mix, then dip into the egg wash. Shake briefly and place onto the frying pan with oil. Cook a few minutes until golden, flip to the other side. Close the lid on the pan and allow the cauliflower pieces to simmer and soften.
5. Remove the fried cauliflower pieces and place onto a paper towel lined plate.
6. Garnish with parsley leaves and serve.

Enjoy!

Keto Edge featured ingredient: CAULIFLOWER

Among health-related properties/actions: Cauliflower is a good source of nutrients, a booster and regulator of digestive health, heart health, inflammation related conditions, researched for cancer-preventive effects.

Among known active molecules/compounds: One of cauliflower antioxidants is indole-3-carbinol, commonly found in cruciferous vegetables and researched for its anticancer properties.

Note: Turmeric, used in this recipe, is absorbed by the body better when it is combined with black pepper. One study's findings suggest that combining cauliflower with curcumin (found in turmeric spice) may help with preventing and treating prostate cancer.

Sources:
Planta Med. 1998, 64(4):353-6.
https://pubmed.ncbi.nlm.nih.gov/9619120
Cancer Lett. 2008, 269(2):291-304.
https://www.ncbi.nlm.nih.gov/pmc/articles/PMC2579766/
Cancer Res. 2006, 66(2):613-21.

Stir-Fried Mushroom & Broccoli
with Coconut and Walnuts

Serves 2

Ingredients

1 cup Baby Bella mushrooms, sliced
1 cup broccoli, chopped
2-4 oz walnuts
1 onion, chopped
2 tbsp olive oil or ghee
1 tbsp lemon juice
1 cup vegetable broth
½ cup coconut cream
¼ tsp Himalayan salt (or to taste)
¼ tsp black pepper (or to taste)

*If you would like to increase the fat content of this meal, 4 strips of cooked crumbled bacon will make a great addition! Note: you can reserve the leftover bacon fat and use it in other recipes.

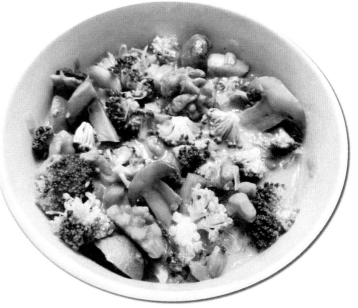

Preparation

1. In a high pan, heat the oil.
2. Add the sliced mushrooms and chopped onions (until onions are slightly golden).
3. Add the vegetable broth and the coconut cream, mix 1-2 min.
4. Add lemon juice, mix briefly.
5. Add the broccoli and walnuts, simmer the mix on low heat for about 10 min until the broccoli is softened.
6. Add salt and pepper and serve.

Enjoy!

Keto Edge featured ingredient: COCONUT CREAM

Among health-related properties/actions: Can help with regulating weight and improving cognition.

Among known active molecules/compounds: Lauric acid (abundant in coconut cream) was shown to have positive effects on cardiovascular and neurological health.

Sources:
J Am Coll Nutr. 2019, 38(2):97-107.
https://pubmed.ncbi.nlm.nih.gov/30395784
J Oleo Sci. 2016, 65(8):693-99.
https://pubmed.ncbi.nlm.nih.gov/27430387
Open Heart. 2016, 3:e000467.
https://openheart.bmj.com/content/3/2/e000467
Biomaterials. 2018, 178:517-26.
https://pubmed.ncbi.nlm.nih.gov/29631784

Roasted Purple Cabbage

Serves 2

Ingredients
1 medium head of purple cabbage, sliced into strips
1 medium onion, chopped
2 oz peeled raw pumpkin seeds
4 tbsp extra virgin olive oil
½ cup vegetable broth
¼ tsp Himalayan salt

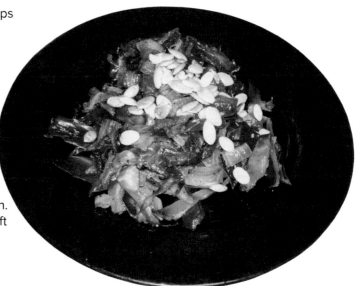

Preparation
1. In a sauté pan, heat the oil.
2. Add the onions and pumpkin seeds, mix 3-4 min.
3. Add the purple cabbage and salt, mix 4-5 min.
4. Add the vegetable broth and simmer until soft (~ 30-35 min), stirring occasionally.

Serve and enjoy!

Keto Edge featured ingredient: ONIONS

Among health-related properties/actions: Immune booster, antioxidant, antimicrobial, supporting cardiovascular health.

Among known active molecules/compounds: Onions contain quercetin, a flavonoid (one category of antioxidant compounds) helpful in eliminating free radicals in the body, helpful in regenerating a powerful antioxidant vit. E, improving endothelial function associated with atherosclerosis thereby improving heart health.

Note: Purple cabbage: rich in antioxidants as well as vitamins A, C, and K.

Sources:
J Am Coll Nutr. 2013, 32(3):160-64.
https://pubmed.ncbi.nlm.nih.gov/23885989
Front Microbiol. 2019, 10:867.
https://www.ncbi.nlm.nih.gov/pmc/articles/PMC6492534/
Article "Onions: Health Benefits, Health Risks & Nutrition Facts." Szalay, J. on LiveScience website.
https://www.livescience.com/45293-onion-nutrition.html
Today's Dietitian. 2018, 20(7):22.
https://www.todaysdietitian.com/newarchives/0718p22.shtml

Sautéed Parsnip Mushrooms

Serves 2

Ingredients

2 medium parsnips, finely chopped
12 oz mushrooms, chopped
1 onion, chopped
¼ cup dill (preferably fresh, or can be dried)
¼ tsp Himalayan salt
¼ tsp black pepper
8 tbsp olive oil
Parsley for garnish

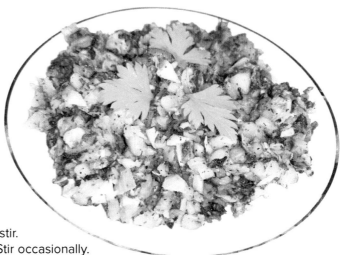

Preparation

1. In a frying pan, heat the oil.
2. Add the mushrooms, onions, and parsnip, stir 4-5 min.
3. Add the spices (dill, salt, black pepper) and stir.
4. Close the lid and cook until all is softened. Stir occasionally. Serve with parsley.

Enjoy!

Keto Edge featured ingredient: DILL

Among health-related properties/actions: Rich in antioxidants, may help with lowering blood sugar, detoxifying foreign compounds, including carcinogens.

Among known active molecules/compounds: D-Limonene is a type of monoterpene, a naturally occurring compound found in dill that was researched in studies to prevent and treat lung, breast, and colon cancer.

Sources:
Herbal Medicine: Biomolecular and Clinical Aspects. Ch.17
https://www.ncbi.nlm.nih.gov/books/NBK92774/
Oncol Rep. 2013, 29(1):349-54.
https://pubmed.ncbi.nlm.nih.gov/23117412-
Onco Targets Ther. 2018, 11:1833–47.
https://www.ncbi.nlm.nih.gov/pmc/articles/PMC5894671/

Brussels Sprouts and Bacon

Serves 2

Ingredients
2 cups Brussels Sprouts, cut in halves
2 strips of bacon, chopped
¼ tsp Himalayan salt
4 tbsp olive oil
Dill for garnish

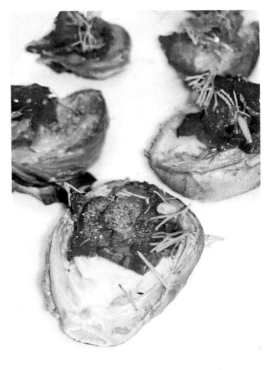

Preparation
1. In a frying pan, add the olive oil with salt and bacon. Heat on medium for 2 min.
2. Add the Brussels Sprouts, mix, and close the lid. Heat on medium for 7-10 min or until the sides of Brussels Sprouts start turning golden.
3. Serve by topping each Brussels Sprout half with bacon pieces. Garnish with dill. Serve warm or chilled.

Enjoy!

Keto Edge featured ingredient: **BRUSSELS SPROUTS**

Among health-related properties/actions: Antioxidant, provide detox support, regulate inflammation, boost immunity, digestive support, cardiovascular support, can aid with maintaining blood sugar levels, may help protect against cancer.

Among known active molecules/compounds: Glucosinolates and isothiocyanates have been shown to reduce the risk of cancers through the induction of detoxification enzymes.

Note: Heat processing of Brussels Sprouts can greatly reduce the concentrations of glucosinolates and isothiocyanates, however their ability to induce the detoxification enzymes in a study with mice was preserved.

Sources:
Article "Brussels Sprouts." On Nutrition Facts.
https://nutritionfacts.org/topics/brussels-sprouts/
Mol Nutr Food Res. 2008, 52(3):330-41.
https://pubmed.ncbi.nlm.nih.gov/18293303
J Food Sci. 2011, 76(3):C454-61.
https://pubmed.ncbi.nlm.nih.gov/21535814

Radicchio Eggplant Ragout

Serves 2-3

Ingredients

1 large eggplant, cut in cubes
1 red bell pepper, chopped
3 tbsp sesame seed oil
3 tbsp olive oil
¼ tsp Himalayan salt
¼ tsp black pepper
4 tbsp lemon juice
1 garlic clove, crushed
Radicchio leaves (or Boston lettuce leaves)
Garnish with sesame seeds and parsley

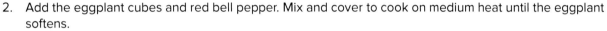

Preparation

1. In a deep frying pan, add the olive oil, garlic, red bell pepper, salt, and black pepper. Briefly mix.
2. Add the eggplant cubes and red bell pepper. Mix and cover to cook on medium heat until the eggplant softens.
3. In a small bowl, mix the sesame oil with lemon juice. Add to the cooked eggplant and briefly mix. Allow to chill.
4. Line the serving plates with Radicchio (or lettuce) leaves and fill with 1-2 tbsp of the eggplant mix. Garnish with sesame seeds, parsley, and serve.

Enjoy!

Keto Edge featured ingredient: RADICCHIO LEAVES

Among health-related properties/actions: Aids with digestion and colon cleansing, antiparasitic, antioxidant, assists with weight loss and maintaining body metabolism, helps with eye health. Among other things, fresh leaves of radicchio are loaded with B-complex vitamins and vitamin K.

Among known active molecules/compounds: Lactucopicrin (intybrin) is an agent that gives radicchio its bitter taste. It is a potent anti-malarial agent with sedative effect and painkiller properties.

Note: Keep in mind that radicchio leaves are distinctly bitter in taste.

Sources:
Article "Health benefits of radicchio." Juicing for Health website.
https://juicing-for-health.com/health-benefits-of-radicchio
J Ethnopharmacol. 2006, 107(2):254-58.
https://pubmed.ncbi.nlm.nih.gov/16621374

desserts

Rich Chocolate Almond Loaf

Pumpkin Pie

Checkerboard Cake

Buttercream Rum Cake

Cranberry Thins

Almond Pecan Cookies

Chocolate Truffles

Dr. Dave's Ice Cream

Rich Chocolate Almond Loaf

Serves 16 (slices)

Ingredients

½ cup whole almonds, coarsely chopped with sharp knife

2 oz or 5-6 squares dark chocolate (90%)

6 tbsp unsalted butter

¾ cup condensed milk (unsweetened)

2 tbsp ground cinnamon

3 oz sugar free amaretti cookies (made of almond flour), broken

½ cup raw cranberries (unsweetened)

1 tsp Stevia sweetener

Preparation

1. Place a sheet of parchment paper in a baking loaf pan (1-lb).
2. In a boiling pan, add the chocolate, butter, condensed milk, and cinnamon. Heat the mixture over low heat for 3-5 min, stirring constantly (use wooden spoon) until the chocolate melts. Add the chopped almonds, broken cookies, and cranberries into the mixture. Stir constantly another 3-4 min.
3. Pour the mixture into the baking pan, cover, let chill, and refrigerate for 1 hour.
4. Cut the loaf into slices and serve.

Enjoy!

Keto Edge featured ingredient: CRANBERRIES

Among health-related properties/actions: Cranberries are a popular superfood. They are known to be used in treating urinary tract infections (UTI), aid with oral health, boost immunity, boost circulation, reduce cardiovascular disease (CVD), support gut health.

Among known active molecules/compounds: Antioxidant proanthocyanidins (PACs) and mannose in cranberries can prevent some bacteria from sticking to the urinary tract walls.

Note: In one study, when cranberry extract was combined with extracts from coconut oil and oregano, it showed eradication of *E.coli* bacteria.

Sources:
Crit Rev Food Sci Nutr. 2002, 42(3 Suppl):273-78.
https://pubmed.ncbi.nlm.nih.gov/12058985
Clin Nutr. 2019, Apr 11.
https://pubmed.ncbi.nlm.nih.gov/31023488
Lett Appl Microbiol. 2019, 68(4):321-28.
https://pubmed.ncbi.nlm.nih.gov/30801748

Pumpkin Pie

Serves 12

Ingredients

Crust:

2 ½ cup almond flour

¼ cup Truvia natural sweetener (or any sweetener of choice; omit for savory pie crust)

¼ tsp Sea salt (or ½ tsp for savory pie crust)

¼ cup coconut oil (measured solid, then melted)

1 large egg

½ tsp vanilla extract (optional)

Filling:

1 15-oz can pumpkin puree

½ cup heavy cream (or coconut cream for dairy-free/paleo)

2 large eggs (at room temperature)

½ cup Truvia natural sweetener

2 tsp pumpkin spice

¼ tsp sea salt

1 tsp vanilla extract (optional)

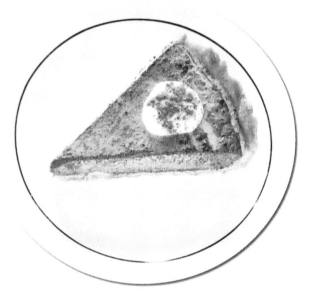

Preparation

1. Preheat the oven to 350°F.
2. Prepare the Crust: In a bowl, mix the crust ingredients and press into a 9-inch form.
3. Bake for 10-12 min. Let cool.
4. Lower the oven temperature to 325°F.
5. Prepare the Filling: In a separate bowl, mix the ingredients for the filling. Pour into a pie crust. Bake for 40-50 min.

Enjoy!

Keto Edge featured ingredient: PUMPKIN

Among health-related properties/actions: Antioxidant, boosts immunity, protects skin, protects eyesight, may benefit heart health and aid in preventing cancer.

Among known active molecules/compounds: Pumpkin is high in carotenoids which help with neutralizing free radicals. The effects are being researched for cancer prevention.

Sources:
Nutr Res Rev. 2010, 23:184-90.
https://pubmed.ncbi.nlm.nih.gov/21110905
Article "Talking Pumpkin with Dr. B." Healthy Aging, Emory University.
https://pubmed.ncbi.nlm.nih.gov/7784309
Pharmacol Res. 1995, 31(1):73-79.
https://pubmed.ncbi.nlm.nih.gov/7784309

Checkerboard Cake

Serves 12

Ingredients

Cake Layers:
½ cup unsalted butter, room temperature
½ cup olive oil
½ cup Truvia natural sweetener
4 eggs, room temperature
1 tbsp vanilla extract
3 cups almond flour
2 tbsp cocoa powder
1 tbsp baking powder
½ tsp salt
1 ¼ cup buttermilk, room temperature

Note: for the checkerboard pattern of the cake layers, use the checkerboard cake pan set (commercially available).

Chocolate Fudge Cream:
6 oz unsweetened dark chocolate, chopped (or 1 cup unsweetened chocolate chips)
1 cup unsalted butter, room temperature
1 cup Truvia natural sweetener
½ tsp vanilla extract
½ tsp salt
2 tbsp heavy cream

Preparation
1. Preheat the oven to 350°F.
2. Prepare two 9-inch round baking pans by lining them with parchment paper.
3. In a large bowl, mix together butter, olive oil and Truvia until creamy and well-integrated.
4. Add one egg at a time, integrating well into the mix after each addition.
5. Stir in vanilla extract.
6. In a separate, medium bowl, whisk together flour, baking powder, and salt.
7. Using a spatula, start adding, interchangeably, the flour mixture and buttermilk to the butter mixture, until fully integrated.
8. Transfer half of the mixture to one of the baking pans. Add the cocoa powder to the remaining batter and mix until integrated. Transfer this half of the mixture to the 2nd 9-inch baking pan. Bake in the oven for 25-30 min. Test with a toothpick (inserted in the center) that no batter sticks to complete the baking.
9. Allow cake layers to cool in their cake pans for 10 min, invert onto cooling racks. When cooled, use the checkerboard cake pan set to cut and interlay the layers for the checkerboard pattern.
10. For the chocolate fudge cream, melt the chocolate in a double-boiler pan, until smooth. Allow to cool until it is tolerably hot.
11. In a separate bowl, place the butter and use a mixer to beat into creamy.
12. Add the cooled chocolate and stir well. Gradually add Truvia while mixing.
13. Add the salt and vanilla extract, stir well.
14. With mixer on low, gradually add heavy cream until fully integrated.
15. Spread the frosting onto prepared, cooled, baked layers. Place in the refrigerator for 30 min or until serving.

Enjoy!

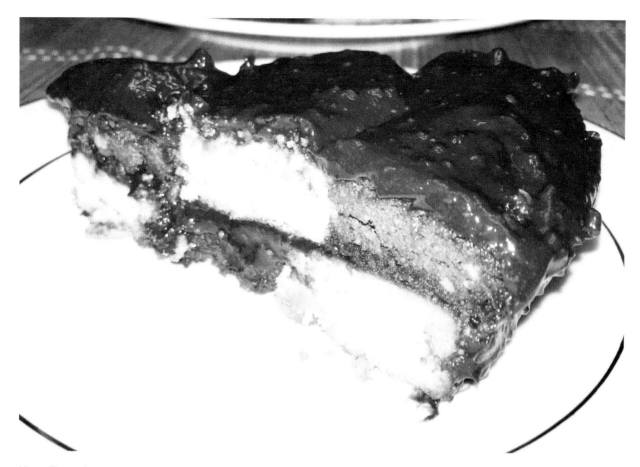

Keto Edge featured ingredient: VANILLA EXTRACT

Among health-related properties/actions: Antioxidant that can be used for food consumption, preservation, and in nutraceuticals; researched in the context of reducing mutation rates, reducing metastatic and invasive properties in cancer cells.

Among known active molecules/compounds: Vanilla extract contains a compound known as vanillin that has antioxidant, antidepressant and antitumor effects.

Note: In a study conducted by Penn State, adding vanilla to milk was shown to make it seem sweeter in taste, suggesting that adding vanilla could help with reducing sugars in a meal.

Sources:
J Agric Food Chem. 2007, 55(19):7738-43.
https://pubmed.ncbi.nlm.nih.gov/17715988
Article by Penn State: "Vanilla makes milk beverages seem sweeter." ScienceDaily. ScienceDaily, 20 June 2019.
https://www.sciencedaily.com/releases/2019/06/190620121410.htm
Oxid Med Cell Longev. 2016, 2016:9734816.
https://www.ncbi.nlm.nih.gov/pmc/articles/PMC5204113/
Mol Cell Biochem. 2018, 438(1-2):35-45.
https://pubmed.ncbi.nlm.nih.gov/28744811

Buttercream Rum Cake

Serves 12
Ingredients

Custard Rum Filling:
¼ cup Truvia natural sweetener
¼ cup cornstarch
¼ tsp salt
2 cups half-and-half
4 large egg yolks
3 tbsp salted butter
2 tbsp rum (or 1 tsp rum extract)

Cake Layers:
1 cup salted butter, softened
1 cup Truvia natural sweetener
4 large eggs
3 ¼ cups almond flour, plus more for dusting pans
2 ½ tsp baking powder
¾ tsp salt
½ tsp ground cinnamon
¼ tsp ground nutmeg
¾ cup whole milk
½ cup heavy cream
1 tsp vanilla extract

Buttercream:
1 cup salted butter, softened
1 tsp vanilla extract
½ cup Truvia natural sweetener
¾-1 cup heavy cream, divided
Grated fresh nutmeg (optional)

Preparation

1. Prepare the Rum Custard Filling: In a boiling pan, whisk together sweetener, cornstarch, and salt.
2. In a separate glass bowl, whisk together half-and-half and egg yolks. Gradually add half-and-half mixture into sweetener mixture. Cook over medium heat, whisking constantly, until mixture starts to bubble, 7-8 min.
3. Remove from heat, add in butter and rum (or rum flavor). Transfer to a medium bowl. Cover (to prevent a film from forming) and let stand 30 min; chill 2-4 hours.
4. Prepare the Cake Layers: Preheat oven to 350°F.
5. Butter mixture: In a bowl, beat the butter with a mixer until creamy. Gradually add the sweetener, until integrated as light and fluffy. Add eggs, one at a time, beating until integrated after each addition.
6. Flour mixture: In a large bowl, stir in the flour, baking powder, salt, cinnamon, and nutmeg.
7. Milk mixture: In a measuring cup, mix whole milk and heavy cream.
8. Add flour mixture to butter mixture alternately with milk mixture (begin and end with flour mixture), until fully integrated after each addition. Mix in vanilla.
9. Prepare 4 9-inch round cake pans, cover with parchment paper. Divide the mass evenly among 4 pans. Bake in preheated oven 15-20 min (test with a wooden pick). Allow to cool.
10. Prepare the Buttercream: Beat the butter with a mixer until creamy. Gradually add vanilla extract and sweetener. Gradually add the ¾ heavy cream mixture, beating on low to high speed until smooth and fluffy. Continue adding up to ¼ cup cream, 1 tablespoon at a time, for desired consistency.
11. Assemble the cake: In a piping bag, place 1 cup of the buttercream. On a serving platter, pipe a 1/2-inch-thick ring of buttercream on the very outer edge of the cake. Spread 1/4 cup of the custard filling inside the ring. Repeat the steps with all layers. Chill 30 min.
12. With the remaining buttercream, choose a favorite icing tip and cover the sides of the cake in a zigzag-like manner, making sure that each zigzag touches the one beside it.
13. If desired, sprinkle cake with nutmeg or additional cinnamon.

Enjoy!

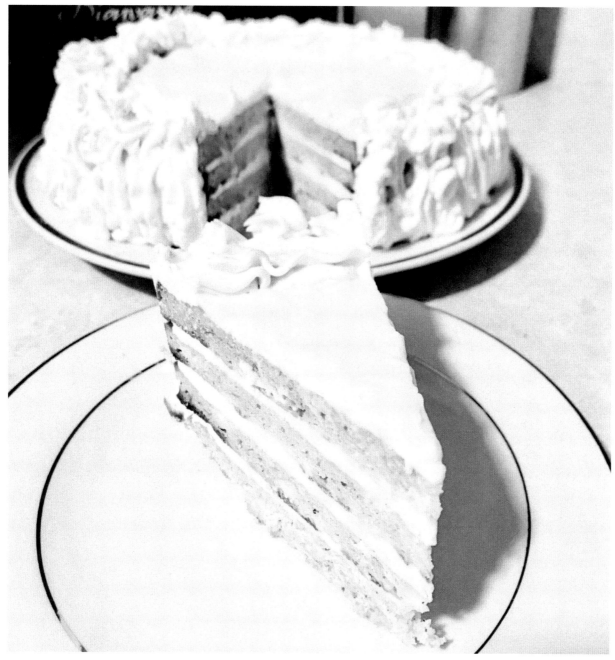

Keto Edge featured ingredient: GROUND CINNAMON
Among health-related properties/actions: Loaded with antioxidants, anti-inflammatory properties, may reduce the risk for heart disease, can reduce insulin resistance, lower blood sugar, lower blood pressure, treat infections.

Among known active molecules/compounds: A compound cinnamaldehyde is thought to be responsible for the metabolic effects observed from cinnamon spice.

Sources:
J Diabetes Sci Technol. 2010, 4(3):685-693.
https://www.ncbi.nlm.nih.gov/pmc/articles/PMC2901047/
Bioimpacts. 2014, 4(2):69-74.
https://www.ncbi.nlm.nih.gov/pmc/articles/PMC4097974/
Food Funct. 2015, 6(3):910-9.
https://pubmed.ncbi.nlm.nih.gov/25629927

Cranberry Thins

Serves 10-12

Ingredients
1 ½ cup almond flour, plus extra for dusting
¾ stick butter, chilled
¼ cup + 2 tsp Truvia natural sweetener
1 large egg
¼ cup dried unsweetened cranberries
1 tsp cardamom powder
1 tsp shredded coconut

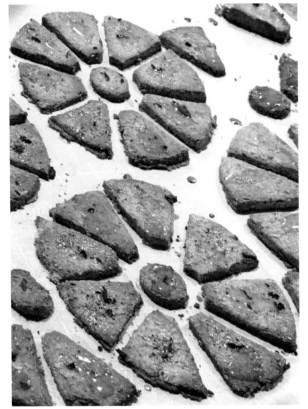

Preparation
1. Preheat the oven to 350°F. Line 1 large cookie sheet with parchment paper.
2. In a bowl, mix the flour with cardamom powder. Add butter and cut to the size of breadcrumbs mix. Add the sweetener (¼ cup).
3. In a separate bowl, whisk the egg lightly and add to the flour mixture.
4. Add the cranberries and mix until the dough forms into a stiff paste.
5. Roll the dough out on a counter, into a ¼ inch thick layer (drizzle with flour as needed). Use the desired cookie cutter shapes and press out the cookies. Transfer the cut pastry to the baking sheets. Bake in the oven for 10-12 min until lightly brown. Allow to cool off.
6. Mix the cold water with the sweetener (2 tsp), the shredded coconut, and drizzle over the cooled cookies. Let stand for 10 min.

Enjoy!

Keto Edge featured ingredient: CARDAMOM POWDER
Among health-related properties/actions: Antioxidant, digestive regulation, diuretic, decongestant, circulatory stimulant, antibacterial, antifungal, anti-inflammatory, oral health, aphrodisiac.

Among known active molecules/compounds: One of the main components in cardamom, gamma-Bisabolene, is researched for its anti-proliferative activities in oral cancer cells in lab.

Sources:
Lipids Health Dis. 2017, 16:151.
https://www.ncbi.nlm.nih.gov/pmc/articles/PMC5557534/
Curr Med Mycol. 2016, 2(2):8-15.
https://pubmed.ncbi.nlm.nih.gov/28681014
Proteomics. 2015, 15(19):3296-309.
https://pubmed.ncbi.nlm.nih.gov/26194454

Almond Pecan Cookies

Serves 10-12

Ingredients

1 cup unsalted butter, softened
½ cup Truvia natural sweetener
1 tsp vanilla extract
2 ½ cups almond flour
¼ teaspoon salt
¾ cup pecan halves

Preparation

1. Preheat oven to 350°F. Line two large baking sheets with parchment paper or bake mats.
2. In a bowl, mix/cream together butter, sweetener, and vanilla extract. Add in the flour and salt until fully combined.
3. Using a 1-tbsp cookie scoop (or measuring tablespoon), scoop out the cookie dough, roll into balls, and top with pecan halves.
4. Place the cookies on the prepared baking sheets. Bake for 14-15 min or until the cookies are set and the bottom is lightly browned. Allow to cool.

Enjoy!

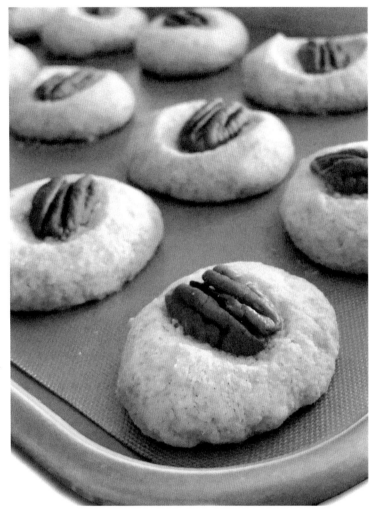

Keto Edge featured ingredient: PECANS

Among health-related properties/actions: Antioxidant, neuroprotective properties, lower the risk of heart disease, regulate cholesterol.

Among known active molecules/compounds: A polyphenol ellagic acid is researched in various cancer cells for its ability to inhibit cell growth.

Sources:
Nutr Res. 2006, 26(8):397-402.
https://www.sciencedirect.com/science/article/pii/S0271531706001278
Ann N Y Acad Sci. 2004, 1031:127-42.
https://pubmed.ncbi.nlm.nih.gov/15753140
Oncotarget. 2017, 8(7):12301-10.
https://www.ncbi.nlm.nih.gov/pmc/articles/PMC5355345/
J Cancer. 2019, 10(15):3303-14.
https://www.ncbi.nlm.nih.gov/pmc/articles/PMC6603400/

Chocolate Truffles

Serves 10-12

Ingredients
8 squares (~ 3 oz) unsweetened dark chocolate (90% cacao)
1 tbsp almond flavoring
3 tbsp unsalted butter
¼ cup of Truvia natural sweetener
4 tbsp cacao powder for rolling

Preparation
1. In a double-boiler pan, melt the chocolate squares and butter. Add the sweetener and the almond flavoring. Mix well.
2. Let the mixture cool until firm (place in a freezer for ~5 min).
3. Use a teaspoon to roll the paste into balls (makes ~24). Place the cacao powder on a flat plate, roll the paste balls to coat them in cacao powder. Place in a freezer for another 5 min and serve.

Enjoy!

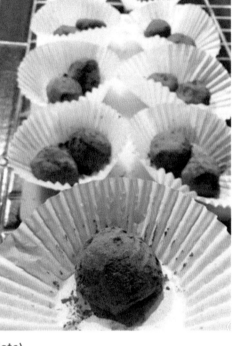

Keto Edge featured ingredient: CACAO POWDER (and dark chocolate)
Among health-related properties/actions: Antioxidant, anti-inflammatory, reduction of blood pressure, improvement of vascular function, regulation of lipid and glucose metabolism.

Among known active molecules/compounds: Cacao is one of the greatest sources of polyphenols such as flavanols, which have potent antioxidant and anti-inflammatory effects, and are researched for anticancer properties.

Note: Cacao powder and chocolate are two products derived from cacao beans. The main difference between cacao and chocolate is the absence or presence of cacao butter. In cacao, cacao butter is little to non-existent. In contrast, chocolate contains cacao butter.

Processing and heating cacao can cause it to lose its beneficial properties. When cacao gets treated with alkaline (to reduce bitterness), it can greatly lower the flavanols.

Consuming organic chocolate (without potential cancer-causing pesticides) is best. With chocolate being acidic (similar to acidic setting that abnormal cells often prefer), it is important to consume in moderation. Chocolate can dehydrate, so remember to hydrate. Balance is key!

Sources:
Food Chem Toxicol. 2013, 56:336-51.
https://pubmed.ncbi.nlm.nih.gov/23439478
Front Nutr. 2017, 4:36.
https://pubmed.ncbi.nlm.nih.gov/28824916
Hypertension. 2012, 60(3):794-801.
https://pubmed.ncbi.nlm.nih.gov/22892813
Article "Cocoa vs Chocolate." DifferenceBetween website.
http://www.differencebetween.net/object/comparisons-of-food-items/difference-between-cocoa-and-chocolate/

Dr. Dave's Black Currant Ice Cream

Serves 5-6

Ingredients

1 quart heavy cream
1 cup black currants, fresh or frozen*
2 tbsp cinnamon
1 tbsp cardamom
1 tsp black sesame oil
2 tbsp lemon juice, if desired
¼ cup Truvia natural sweetener or equivalent Stevia

* This recipe works with any berry. We have used blueberries, strawberries, raspberries, mulberries. Just make sure to check the portion size in terms of how much you use for carbohydrate counts.

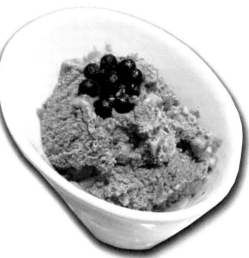

Preparation

1. In a NutriBullet or a similar mixer, mix 1 cup of frozen fruit with half of the cream (0.5 quart) and all of the sweetener. Pour into frozen container from Cuisinart ice cream maker. Start the machine.
2. Add the rest of the cream. Add cinnamon, cardamom, black sesame oil, and lemon juice. Once mixed, sample to sweeten with Truvia. Mix ~20 min. to insure adequate mixing.
3. Stop the machine, transfer the soft ice cream mixture into serving containers and freeze deeper in the freezer, or serve soft.
4. Garnish with berries.

Enjoy the smooth delicious taste!

Keto Edge featured ingredient: **BLACK CURRANT**

Among health-related properties/actions: Boosts immunity, regulates blood pressure, exhibits both antiviral and antibacterial properties; antioxidant and antiproliferative properties.

Among known active molecules/compounds: Dietary antioxidants from black currant, such as anthocyanins, are researched in lab for their chemopreventive properties with liver cancer mentioned as an example.

Sources:
Microbiol Immunol. 2012, 56(12):805-09.
https://pubmed.ncbi.nlm.nih.gov/22985050
Nat Prod Commun. 2010, 5(10):1613-18.
https://pubmed.ncbi.nlm.nih.gov/21121259
J Nutr Biochem. 2011, 22(11):1035-46.
https://pubmed.ncbi.nlm.nih.gov/21216582

Made in the USA
Middletown, DE
04 October 2022

11924525R00062